Diabetes
CARB
CONTROL
Cookbook

Director, Book Publishing, Abe Ogden; Managing Editor, Greg Guthrie; Acquisitions Editor, Victor Van Beuren; Editor, Rebekah Renshaw; Production Manager, Melissa Sprott; Composition, Circle Graphics; Cover Design, pixiedesign, llc; Photographer, Kelly Campbell; Printer, Versa Press.

Printed in the United States of America
1 3 5 7 9 10 8 6 4 2

The suggestions and information contained in this publication are generally consistent with the Clinical Practice Recommendations and other policies of the American Diabetes Association, but they do not represent the policy or position of the Association or any of its boards or committees. Reasonable steps have been taken to ensure the accuracy of the information presented. However, the American Diabetes Association cannot ensure the safety or efficacy of any product or service described in this publication. Individuals are advised to consult a physician or other appropriate health care professional before undertaking any diet or exercise program or taking any medication referred to in this publication. Professionals must use and apply their own professional judgment, experience, and training and should not rely solely on the information contained in this publication before prescribing any diet, exercise, or medication. The American Diabetes Association—its officers, directors, employees, volunteers, and members—assumes no responsibility or liability for personal or other injury, loss, or damage that may result from the suggestions or information in this publication.

⊗ The paper in this publication meets the requirements of the ANSI Standard Z39.48-1992 (permanence of paper).

ADA titles may be purchased for business or promotional use or for special sales. To purchase more than 50 copies of this book at a discount, or for custom editions of this book with your logo, contact the American Diabetes Association at the address below, at booksales@diabetes.org, or by calling 703-299-2046.

American Diabetes Association
1701 North Beauregard Street
Alexandria, Virginia 22311
DOI: 10.2337/9781580405171

Library of Congress Cataloging-in-Publication Data

Hughes, Nancy S.
  Diabetes carb control cookbook / Nancy S. Hughes.
     pages cm
  Summary: "This easy-fix, easy-to-follow cookbook contains 150 recipes with the same amount of carbohydrates in every single recipe . . . only 15 grams of carbohydrates in each"—Provided by publisher.
  Includes bibliographical references and index.
  ISBN 978-1-58040-517-1 (paperback)
  1. Diabetes—Diet therapy—Recipes. I. Title.
  RC662.H8354 2014
  641.5'6314—dc23
              2014008264

Diabetes
CARB
CONTROL
Cookbook

NANCY S. HUGHES

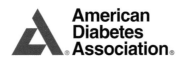

American Diabetes Association.

Dedication

To my children: Will, Annie, and Taft; their spouses: Kelly, Terry, and Kara; and to my grandchildren: Molly Catherine, Anna Flynn, Jilli, Jesse, and Emma. The refrigerators were bulging, tastings were constant, and you never knew what to expect when you walked into the kitchen . . . except one thing: a tight squeeze from me every single time. You make me happier than you'll ever imagine.

To my husband, Greg: You are a true sport! You deal with the chaos, the commotion, the craziness of my "dither days," and since you obviously know how happy it makes me, you just take a deep breath and hold on! Thanks for holding on . . . so tight!!

It's fun, isn't it!

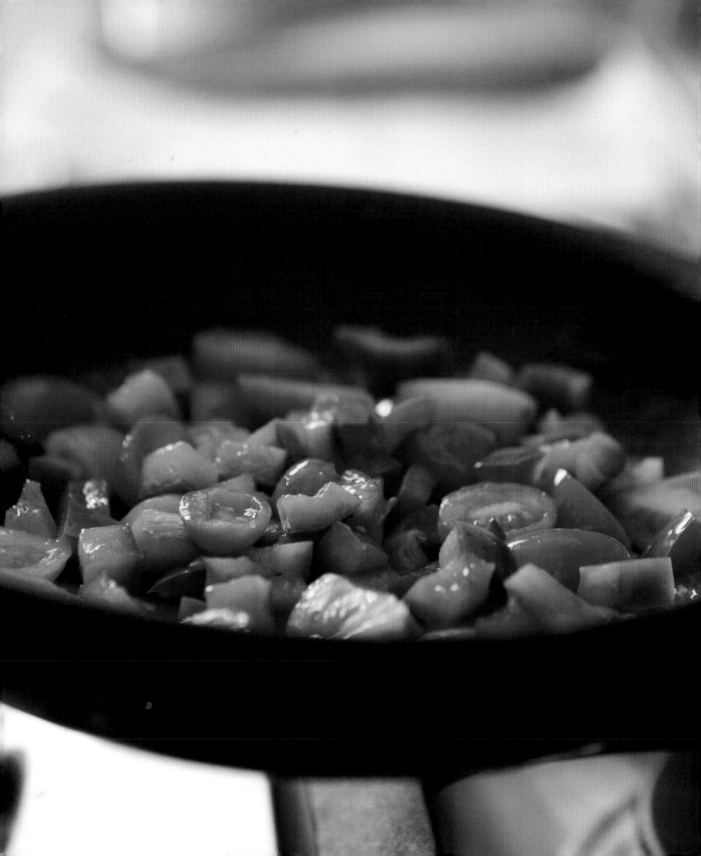

Acknowledgments

To Melanie McKibbin, my business manager, who kept me organized, took my piles of "to do" lists and did them herself (sometimes voluntarily), and knew when to transform what I was trying to say into complete sentences.

To Sylvia Vollmer, my very positive, very conscientious assistant, who learned to read my chicken scratch, read my mind, and thoroughly enjoy every taste test, no matter what time it was or how many tastings were conducted that day.

To Abe Ogden, Director of Book Publishing; Victor VanBeuren, Acquisitions Editor; and Rebekah Renshaw, my go-to-for-everything editor, thank you for being there for me . . . always, always.

I love what I do and you definitely are a part of that fun!

—Nancy S. Hughes

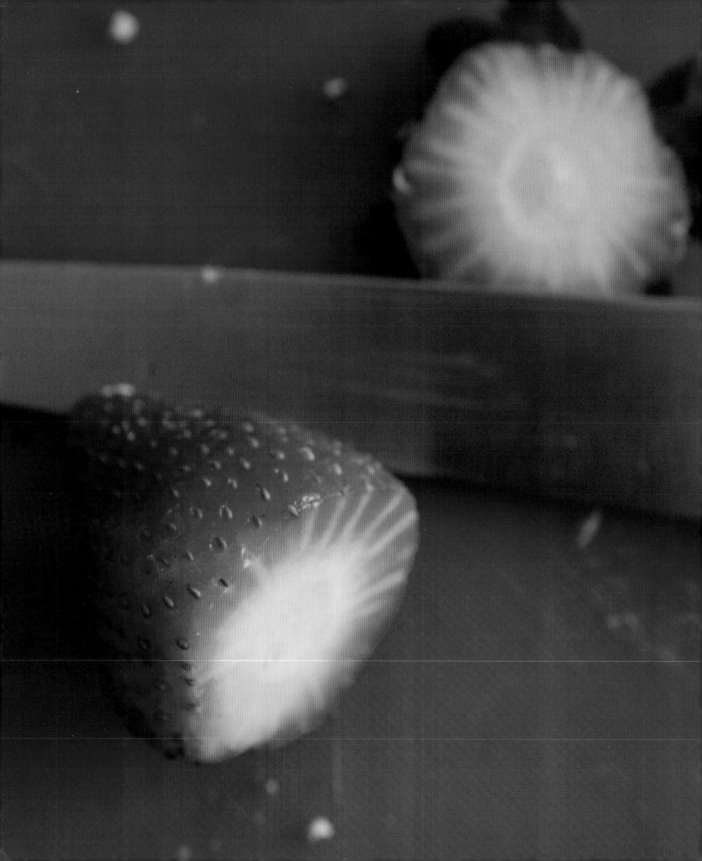

Preface

As I've grown through the years, I've come to realize that the simpler things are, the happier and calmer I am. That's the way I hope you feel about my books. You can rely on my recipes being easy and simple, which, in turn, makes your lives happier and calmer.

I hope you agree!

Enjoy!

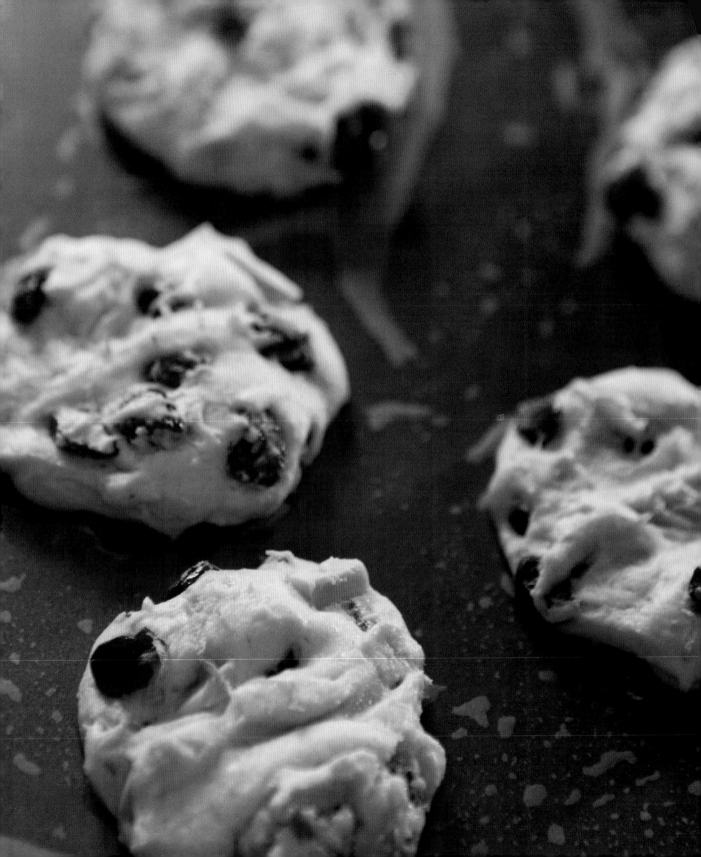

Table of Contents

15-Gram Carbohydrate Recipes for People with Diabetes

(Carb-controlled recipes for breakfast, lunch, dinner, snacks, and dessert containing 15 grams of carbohydrates per serving)

This easy-fix, easy-to-follow cookbook contains 150 recipes with the same amount of carbohydrates in every single recipe . . . only 15 grams of carbohydrates or LESS in each!

This book is a great tool to help portion control and control the intake of carbs. It's important for people with diabetes to keep up with the amount of carbohydrates they consume, but it can be a confusing task. Life brings on many demands. Adding one more, even though it's important, can be overwhelming.

Consistency, on the other hand, brings a sense of calm in a stressful world. It also brings a sense of "sensibility" by controlling food portions and having absolutely no question of the amount of carbs consumed!

Cookbooks for people with diabetes have helpful recipes that always include the amount of carbohydrates per serving. But this cookbook goes one step further and offers *uniformity* in carbohydrate content. This means all the recipes have the same amount of carbs no matter what recipe you choose to make in the entire book!

Carbohydrate foods are a very important part of good nutrition, but it is the carbohydrate in foods that raise your blood sugar the most. All carbohydrates, no matter what the source, can raise your blood glucose if you eat too much at one time. *Counting* carbohydrates can help you gain better control of your blood sugar levels; *spacing* your carbohydrate foods throughout the day helps to control your blood glucose levels, too.

In this book, you will also find a listing of alternative 15-gram carb choices for those days when a "plain-and-basic" food option is all that's needed. This will help you have even more choices and keep you on track . . . easily! Be sure to keep some of these items on hand at all times to fall back on at the end of a busy day.

As with all of my books, my goal is to provide easy-to-make recipes with familiar ingredients that you can find in your local grocery store. Cook's tips, helpful short-cut techniques, total yields, and serving size amounts will make you feel at ease . . . and informed. The recipes are easy and packed with flavor with easily obtainable, familiar ingredients to please the entire family.

I wanted to give you a tool to use that will bring some calm into your life and enjoyment to your meals . . . again! "Hope you're hungry!!"—Nancy S. Hughes

It's All About the Stretch!

So how can you enjoy the carbs you've always loved and stay on track?
. . . the secret's in the stretch!

Trick your taste buds *and* your eyes by incorporating higher-carb ingredients with lower carbs. You'll get that satisfying feeling that comes from higher-carb ingredients without "over-carbing" when you add bulk with the lower carbs! This mixing of carbs opens up a whole new chapter of food combinations that pop with color, texture, flavor, and "carb" fulfillment! Not only are you controlling your carbs in this cookbook, but you are increasing your vegetable and fruit intake!

S-T-R-E-T-C-H-I-N-G TECHNIQUES

Bulk It Up:
- Add veggies (sautéed or tossed in during the last few minutes of cooking) to your rice and pasta dishes. You're still getting the starches you love, but the serving size is larger without going overboard.

- Stretching your higher-carb foods really opens fun, flavor-filled combinations. Instead of a simple small side of boiled potatoes, why not toss those potatoes with sautéed mushrooms, onions, and garlic in a bit of olive oil? Little effort for great flavor!
- You can still have your rice, your pasta, and your bread. It's the amount that you need to control and the type that you buy. When purchasing these ingredients, it's important to look for ones with higher fiber content. These are the whole-grain variety. Read the labels. You're looking for the fiber content. The higher the fiber, the better it is for you. Also, when combining these ingredients with other higher-fiber items, such as low carb veggies, it raises the overall fiber content of the dish considerably. Keep in mind, even though these carbs are a good source of fiber, you still have to be careful how much you consume, so combine them with lower-carb veggies and lean protein to get the most out of your meals.

Give Body and Balance:

- When making salads, for example, try tossing small amounts of higher-carb ingredients, such as whole grains like bulgur, brown rice, or even corn with lower-carb veggies for a more substantially satisfying salad.
- Add meaty veggies to your entree to make it feel and taste heartier, such as mushrooms, grape tomatoes, or carrots.

Camouflage It:

- Cook diced sweet potatoes with diced carrots, for example, to give the taste and texture of sweet potatoes with only a fraction of the carbs!

- Add cauliflower to your favorite pasta and potato salads. Add the cauliflower to the pasta or potatoes during the last few minutes of cooking. It gives the "feel" of pasta or potatoes and it absorbs the flavors of the other ingredients, much like potatoes and pastas do.

Pasta Stand-Ins:
- Get more of a "spaghetti noodle" feel by incorporating "zucchini ribbons" into your pasta dish! Using a vegetable peeler, cut in long strips down the length of the zucchini to form "ribbons." Pop them in the boiling water during the last 15 seconds of cooking.
- When serving spaghetti noodles, thinly slice bell peppers lengthwise to give them a "noodle" type feel. If serving penne or rotini pasta, cut the peppers, or veggies such as zucchini or carrots, in 2-inch strips to blend with the shape of the pasta.

It's In the Cut:
- Use a serrated knife and cut your bread a little thinner to feel like more! Rub it with a halved clove of garlic and sprinkle with fresh herbs for a fat-free, high-flavored addition.
- Make your dishes feel more satisfying by incorporating chunkier pieces of lean protein and vegetables into your dishes. Instead of finely chopping an ingredient, try coarsely chopping for a heartier taste.

Show It Off:
- Top stuffed peppers or a mushroom entrée with toasted bread crumbs. Don't "stuff" it with the bread crumbs . . . "accent"

with them! That way you will know, taste, and *see* what you're getting, instead of the breadcrumbs getting lost inside.

- Top your salads with homemade croutons, preferably the whole grain variety. Simply cut a bread slice into ½-inch cubes and toast in a 350°F oven for 10 minutes, let cool before serving.

Think Outside the Bread Box

- Don't eat with your fingers! Not every sandwich has to be hand-held. What's wrong with the knife and fork approach? It makes a sandwich feel more special . . . with half the carbs! When you pile the ingredients up high, it not only looks inviting, it feels like you're eating a lot . . . and you are! A lot of high-flavored, high-textured veggies.
- Rethink the handheld sandwich! Fill long romaine leaves with your favorite sandwich fillers. Eat it as you would a burrito or hot dog. The long leaves are fun to eat, too!

Change Up the Bases:

- Be adventurous with your snacks and appetizers. Crackers are great for bases, but what about branching out and using other bases that bring interest, crunch, and freshness to a dish, such as thick cucumber slices, Belgian endive leaves, and even rounds of plum tomatoes. They're all extremely low in carbs, too!

Plain & Basic

When you just need some "plain-and-basic" items to go along with your other dishes, here are some suggestions. These will help keep things simple, but keep you on track. If you can stock up on some of these ingredients, it will be extremely helpful, especially when you are out of time and need a quick double dish!

10 SIMPLE SEASONINGS

1. Fresh lemon or lime juice
2. Buttery spray or olive oil
3. Hot pepper sauce
4. Salt-free seasoning blends
5. Dried herbs or ground spices
6. Chopped fresh herbs
7. Grated citrus zest, such as lemon, orange, or lime
8. Grated fresh ginger
9. Minced fresh garlic
10. Sugar substitute

ALTERNATIVE 15 GRAM CARB CHOICES

Breads

½ whole-grain bagel

1 whole-grain *mini* bagel

½ whole-grain English muffin

1½ slices *reduced calorie* whole-grain bread

1 slice or 1 ounce regular whole-grain bread

1 slice (1 oz) raisin bread

1 biscuit (2½-inch diameter)

1 reduced-fat waffle (4½ inches square)

2 crisp breadsticks (4-inch long × ½-inch in diameter)

6-inch corn tortilla

7-inch low-carb high-fiber flour tortilla

1-ounce slice French or Italian bread

1 small white or whole-grain roll (1 oz)

1 (2-inch) piece cornbread (1½ oz)

Cereals and Grains

⅓ cup bran cereal

½ cup unsweetened, ready-to-eat cereal

½ cup cooked grits

½ cup cooked oatmeal

3 tablespoons low-fat granola

½ cup cooked bulgur

⅓ cup regular or whole-wheat couscous

½ cup cooked regular or whole-grain pasta

½ cup cooked quinoa

½ cup cooked bulgur

⅓ cup cooked brown or white rice

Starchy Vegetables

½ cup corn kernels

1 medium corn on the cob (5 oz)

3 ounces white or sweet potato

1 cup acorn or butternut squash cubes

¾ cup cooked beet slices

Beans, Peas, Lentils

¾ cup shelled edamame

⅓ cup beans, such as garbanzo, pinto, kidney, white, lima, and black-eyed peas

⅔ cup peas, such as green peas

½ cup cooked lentils

Snack Crackers/Chips

3 graham crackers (2½-inch squares each)

4 melba toast slices

21 oyster crackers

2⅔ cups no-fat or low-fat popcorn

¾ ounce pretzels

15–20 fat-free tortilla chips (¾ oz total)

15–20 fat-free potato chips (¾ oz total)

7 whole-wheat crackers (1 oz total)

5 reduced-fat crackers, such as Triscuit

12 small reduced-fat wheat crackers, such as Wheat Thins

24 cheese-flavored crackers, such as Cheezits

2 slices crispbread, such as Wasa

Fruit

1 small apple (4 oz)

1 cup sliced apples

½ cup unsweetened applesauce

4 whole fresh apricots (5½ oz total)

½ cup canned apricot

½ cup banana slices

¾ cup blackberries

¾ cup blueberries

1 cup melon cubes, such as cantaloupe and honeydew

½ cup sweet, fresh cherries

2 medium fresh figs

½ cup fruit cocktail

½ large grapefruit

¾ cup grapefruit sections

½ cup grapes

1 kiwi

¾ cup mandarin oranges
½ cup chopped mango
1 small nectarine (5 oz)
1 cup papaya cubes
1 medium peach (6 oz)
½ cup canned peaches
½ of a large pear (4 oz)
¾ cup chopped fresh pineapple

½ cup canned pineapple
2 small plums (5 oz total)
½ cup canned plums
1 cup raspberries
1¼ cups whole strawberries
2 small tangerines (8 oz total)
1¼ cups watermelon cubes

Dried Fruits

3 dates or prunes
7 dried apricot halves
1½ dried figs

2 tablespoons dried fruit, such
   as raisins, (reduced sugar
   and regular) cranberries,
   and cherries

Fruit Juices

(Note: There's not as much fiber in juice as there is in the actual fruit)

½ cup apple juice
⅓ cup cranberry juice cocktail
1 cup reduced-calorie cranberry
   juice cocktail
⅓ cup fruit juice blends
   (100% juice)

⅓ cup grape juice
½ cup grapefruit juice
½ cup orange juice
½ cup pineapple juice
⅓ cup prune juice

Dairy

1 cup fat-free or low-fat milk
¾ cup plain nonfat or
   low-fat yogurt or Greek
   yogurt

1 cup nonfat or low-fat fruit-
   flavored yogurt sweetened
   with sugar substitute
1 cup fat-free or low-fat buttermilk

Dessert/Snack

2-inch square brownie, unfrosted

2-inch square cake, unfrosted

2 small fat-free cookies

2 small sandwich cookies with
   crème filling

1 frozen fruit juice bar (100% juice)

3 gingersnaps

5 vanilla wafers

1 granola bar (not fat-free)

⅓ cup light ice cream

⅓ cup fat-free or low-fat frozen
   yogurt

½ cup sugar-free, low-fat
   pudding

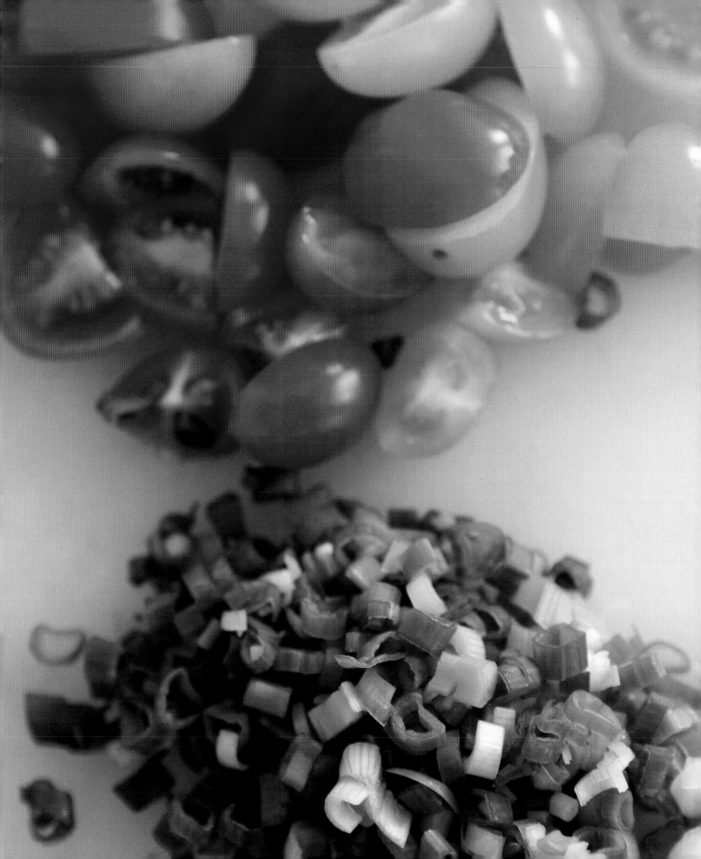

Carb Counting and Meal Planning

To be successful in maintaining a healthy diet and managing your diabetes, you have to start with a plan. A meal plan is an invaluable tool that can help you plan, shop for, and cook healthy meals that fit your lifestyle, schedule, tastes, and health needs. With the right meal plan, you can improve your blood glucose, manage your weight, and even improve your cholesterol and blood pressure.

Meal planning has several additional benefits besides helping you manage your blood glucose. By planning your meals for an entire week, you can make a master shopping list and save time by going to the grocery store just once. You'll also save money by cooking at home more often and cutting down on food waste, and reduce the stress of the five o'clock "what's for dinner" dilemma. Meal planning can help you eat healthier as you plan ahead for healthy meals and avoid relying on convenience products and fast food.

So how do you get started with meal planning? Set aside a specific time when you will plan your meals each week. Set yourself up for success by choosing practical meals that will fit into your schedule. Then make a grocery list and do all of your shopping for the week in one trip.

It's important for people with diabetes to balance the amount of carbohydrates in the food they eat with insulin, medication, and exercise to keep their blood glucose level in a healthy range. Carbohydrate counting helps you keep track of the amount of carbohydrates you eat and space them throughout the day for the best blood glucose control. Maintaining consistency in the grams of carbohydrate you eat from day to day at a given meal is an easy way to help simplify the goal of matching the amount of carbohydrate you eat with insulin, medication, and exercise.

As someone with diabetes, remember to consider carbohydrate counting when creating your meal plan. The amount of carbohydrate you need at each meal can vary depending on your medications and your activity level. Counting carbs is easy with this cookbook because every recipe contains the same amount of carbohydrate – 15 grams. We've provided a sample meal plan here to help you get started. You may need more or less carbohydrate at each meal. Your doctor or dietitian can help you adjust your meal plan and figure out the right amount of carbohydrate for you to help you control your blood glucose.

- **Breakfast:** 30 grams carbohydrate
- **Snack:** 15 grams carbohydrate
- **Lunch:** 45 grams carbohydrate
- **Snack:** 15 grams carbohydrate
- **Dinner:** 45 grams carbohydrate
- **Dessert:** 15 grams carbohydrate

MONDAY

- **Breakfast:** Peanut Butter and Banana Toasters; Purple Swirl Smoothie
- **Snack:** 12 small reduced-fat wheat crackers and 1 (0.75-oz) light cheese snack
- **Lunch:** Tomato-Cilantro Soup; Layered Chicken Taco Salad; 2 small tangerines
- **Snack:** Sweet-Hot Pepper Relish on Cream Cheese
- **Dinner:** Cajun Chicken Stew; ⅓ cup cooked brown rice; Hearty Skillet Kale
- **Dessert:** Peanut Butter and Chocolate Chip Frozen Yogurt

TUESDAY

- Breakfast: Quiche in a Cup; 1 whole grain mini bagel with 1 teaspoon diet margarine
- Snack: Yogurt with Syrup'd Strawberries and Almonds
- Lunch: Protein Hummus and Crisp Veggies; Pear-Cucumber Mint Salad; 7 whole wheat crackers (or pita chips)
- Snack: 1 granola bar (not fat-free)
- Dinner: Beef and Corn-Stuffed Skillet Peppers; Black Bean and Romaine Salad; Spicy Cheddar Broccoli Rice
- Dessert: Pomegranate Peach Ice

WEDNESDAY

- Breakfast: Lemon-Strawberry Oatmeal; 1 cup fat-free or low-fat milk
- Snack: Apples with Creamy Chocolate Peanut Butter Dip

- Lunch: Chicken and Toasted Pecan Salad; 4 slices melba toast; ½ large pear
- Snack: 4-oz cup low-fat cottage cheese with ⅓ cup canned pineapple and dash cinnamon
- Dinner: Saucy Chicken and Peppers; Sneaky Mashed Potatoes; Herbed Panko Asparagus Spears
- Dessert: Brownie Bites

THURSDAY

- Breakfast: Ham and Cream Cheese English Muffins; Raspberry Lemon Honeydew
- Snack: Nutty, Seedy Cereal Snack Mix
- Lunch: Deviled Egg Salad Pitas; 1 small apple; ¾ oz fat-free potato chips
- Snack: Jalapeno-Sour Cream Dip and Raw Veggies
- Dinner: Cod with Avocado Corn Salsa; Black Beans and Tomato with Lime; 1 (6-inch) corn tortilla
- Dessert: Blueberry-Lemon Cupcakers

FRIDAY

- Breakfast: Banana and Toasted Pecan Bread; 1 cup nonfat or low-fat fruit-flavored yogurt w/ sugar substitute
- Snack: 2 small plums with 12 almonds
- Lunch: Ham-Swiss on Rye with Creamy Coleslaw Topping; ¾ oz pretzels; ½ cup grapes
- Snack: Bulgur, Mint, and Tomatoes on Cucumber Rounds

- Dinner: Eggplant-Basil Rounds; Rosemary Garlic Multi Grain Bread; Parmesan Garlic Spinach
- Dessert: Cereal Cookie Rounds

SATURDAY

- Breakfast: Huevos Rancheros; Creamy Grits with Sautéed Green Chiles
- Snack: Fresh Nectarine-Kiwi Salad
- Lunch: Sausage, Bean, and Carrot Soup; Feta-Basil Crostini; 1 cup melon cubes
- Snack: Easy Poppin' Lemon-Dill Popcorn
- Dinner: Sweet Pea and Bacon Salad; Creamy Curried Chicken and Broccoli; ½ cup unsweetened applesauce
- Dessert: Apple Pie Phyllo Tarts

SUNDAY

- Breakfast: Ham and Potato Skillet Quiche; Mighty Tomato Juice
- Snack: ¾ cup watermelon cubes with 2 tablespoons goat cheese and 1 teaspoon honey
- Lunch: Knife and Fork Beefy Corn Tortilla Pies; Lime'd Edamame and Avocado Salad; ½ cup chopped mango
- Snack: Herbed Tomato-Olive Relish with Pita Chips
- Dinner: Beef Sirloin with Shallot-Mushroom Sauce; ½ cup cooked grits or polenta; Baked Tomatoes with Panko and Parmesan
- Dessert: Toffee Almond Poached Pears

Breakfast

BREAD AND CEREAL DISHES

Breakfast Pork and Green Chili Wraps

Minute Breakfast Tortilla Flats

Ham and Cream Cheese English Muffins

Raspberry-Ginger French Toast

Banana and Toasted Pecan Bread

Peanut Butter and Banana Toasters

Lemon-Strawberry Oatmeal

Creamy Grits with Sauteed Chilies

Tomato, Bacon, and Cheddar Grits

FRUITS AND YOGURTS

Buttery Orange and Hot Apple Slices

Raspberry Lemon Honeydew

Yogurt with Syrup'd Strawberries
    and Almonds

Citrus Blueberry Yogurt Bowls

EGG DISHES AND MORE

Quiche in a Cup
Ham and Potato Skillet Quiche
Baked Spinach-Bacon Casserole
Lemon Asparagus Panko Frittata
Huevos Rancheros
Poached Eggs on Chopped Toast
Creamed Eggs on Toast
Open-Faced Egg Sandwiches
Skillet Chicken Sausage with Potatoes

JUICES AND SMOOTHIES

Strawberry Power Juicer or Slush
Mighty Tomato Juice
Purple Swirl Smoothie
Creamy Peanutty Chiller

Breakfast Pork and Green Chili Wraps

SERVES: 4 / **SERVING SIZE:** 1 tortilla, 3 ounces cooked pork, and ¼ cup tomato mixture

1 pound center-cut pork chops, trimmed and thinly sliced
½ teaspoon ground cumin
¼ teaspoon salt
   Black pepper, to taste
1 tablespoon extra-virgin olive oil, divided use
4 low-carb, high-fiber flour tortillas, such as La Tortilla Factory, warmed
1 cup diced tomatoes or grape tomatoes, quartered
1 (4.5-ounce) can chopped mild green chilies
½ cup fat-free sour cream
¼ cup chopped cilantro
1 medium lime, quartered (optional)

1. Sprinkle the pork with the cumin, salt, and pepper. Heat 1 teaspoon of the oil in a large skillet over high heat. Cook the pork 3–4 minutes or until slightly pink in center, stirring frequently. Place a tortilla on each of 4 dinner plates. Spoon equal amounts of the pork on top of each tortilla.

2. To pan residue in skillet: add the tomatoes and the green chilies and cook 2 minutes or until tomatoes are just tender. Remove from heat.

3. Stir in remaining 2 teaspoons oil, spoon over pork, and top with sour cream and cilantro. Serve with lime wedges, if desired.

EXCHANGES/CHOICES
1½ starch, 4 lean meat, ½ fat

Calories	270	**Potassium**	610 mg
Calories from Fat	100	**Total Carbohydrate**	15 g
Total Fat	12 g	Dietary Fiber	8 g
Saturated Fat	2.5 g	Sugars	2 g
Trans Fat	0 g	**Protein**	31 g
Cholesterol	75 mg	**Phosphorus**	300 mg
Sodium	410 mg		

Minute Breakfast Tortilla Flats

SERVES: 4 / **SERVING SIZE:** 1 tortilla

1 Working with one tortilla at a time, place a corn tortilla on a microwave-safe plate. Spread 1 tablespoon of the green chilies on the tortilla, sprinkle with 2 tablespoons of the tomatoes, a small amount of pepper flakes, ¼ cup ham, and 2 tablespoons cheese.

2 Cook in microwave on high setting for 1 minute or until cheese is melted slightly. Remove from microwave and let stand 1 minute.

3 Repeat with remaining tortillas and ingredients.

- **4** soft corn tortillas
- **½** (4.5-ounce) can chopped mild green chilies
- **½** cup grape tomatoes, quartered
- **¼** teaspoon dried red pepper flakes (optional)
- **4** ounces extra-lean diced ham
- **2** ounces shredded part-skim mozzarella

EXCHANGES/CHOICES
1 starch, 1½ lean meat

Calories	140	**Potassium**	190 mg
Calories from Fat	45	**Total Carbohydrate**	13 g
Total Fat	5 g	Dietary Fiber	2 g
Saturated Fat	2 g	Sugars	2 g
Trans Fat	0 g	**Protein**	11 g
Cholesterol	25 mg	**Phosphorus**	200 mg
Sodium	440 mg		

Ham and Cream Cheese English Muffins

SERVES: 4 / **SERVING SIZE:** 1 muffin

2 whole-wheat English muffins, halved

4 ounces diced lower-sodium extra-lean ham

¼ cup light cream cheese

2 tablespoons finely chopped green onion

½ cup grape tomatoes, quartered

 Preheat broiler.

 Place the muffin halves on a baking sheet and broil 1–2 minutes or until just beginning to lightly brown, watching carefully so it doesn't burn.

3 Meanwhile, in a small bowl, combine the ham, cream cheese, and green onion.

4 Spoon equal amounts on each of the muffin halves, top with the tomatoes, and broil 2 minutes or until tomatoes begin to blister slightly.

EXCHANGES/CHOICES
1 starch, 1 lean meat, ½ fat

Calories	140	**Potassium**	250 mg
Calories from Fat	45	**Total Carbohydrate**	15 g
Total Fat	5 g	Dietary Fiber	3 g
Saturated Fat	2 g	Sugars	4 g
Trans Fat	0 g	**Protein**	10 g
Cholesterol	25 mg	**Phosphorus**	180 mg
Sodium	470 mg		

Raspberry-Ginger French Toast

SERVES: 4 / **SERVING SIZE:** 1 bread slice with 3 tablespoons berry mixture and 2 tablespoons yogurt

1. Gently stir together the raspberries, sugar substitute, and ginger in a small bowl. Set aside.

2. Heat the oil in a large nonstick skillet over medium heat.

3. Place the eggs and water in a 13 × 9-inch baking dish. Whisk until well blended. Place the bread slices in the egg mixture and turn several times to coat evenly.

4. Cook the bread slices in the skillet for 3 minutes on each side or until golden.

5. Top each with equal amounts of berry mixture and yogurt.

¾	cup fresh or frozen, thawed raspberries
1	tablespoon Splenda sugar substitute
½	teaspoon grated ginger (optional)
1	tablespoon canola oil
4	large eggs, beaten
2	tablespoons water
4	reduced-calorie whole-wheat bread slices
½	cup nonfat, plain Greek yogurt

EXCHANGES/CHOICES
1 starch, 1½ lean meat, 1 fat

Calories	180	**Potassium**	180 mg
Calories from Fat	80	**Total Carbohydrate**	15 g
Total Fat	9 g	Dietary Fiber	4 g
Saturated Fat	2 g	Sugars	3 g
Trans Fat	0 g	**Protein**	13 g
Cholesterol	190 mg	**Phosphorus**	180 mg
Sodium	160 mg		

Banana and Toasted Pecan Bread

SERVES: 16 / **SERVING SIZE:** ½-inch slice

1⅓ cups white whole-wheat flour
1 teaspoon baking powder
1 teaspoon baking soda
¼ teaspoon salt
¼ cup packed brown sugar substitute blend
3 ounces chopped pecan pieces, toasted
3 ripe medium bananas, mashed (1½ cups mashed)
¼ cup canola oil
¼ cup egg substitute
¼ cup water
1 teaspoon vanilla, butter, and nut flavoring or 1½ teaspoons vanilla extract
1 tablespoon flaxseed meal

1 Preheat oven to 350°F.

2 Whisk together the flour, baking powder, baking soda, and salt in a large bowl. Whisk in the sugar and pecans.

3 Whisk together the remaining ingredients, except the flaxseed meal, in a medium bowl. Stir into the dry ingredients until just blended. Do not overmix.

4 Pour batter into a 9 × 5 × 3-inch nonstick loaf pan coated with cooking spray. Sprinkle evenly with the flaxseed meal. Bake for 50 minutes or until a wooden pick inserted in center comes out clean. Cool in pan on a wire rack 10 minutes; remove from pan, and cool completely on wire rack.

EXCHANGES/CHOICES
1 starch, 1½ fat

Calories	140	**Potassium**	120 mg
Calories from Fat	70	**Total Carbohydrate**	15 g
Total Fat	8 g	Dietary Fiber	3 g
Saturated Fat	0.5 g	Sugars	4 g
Trans Fat	0 g	**Protein**	3 g
Cholesterol	0 mg	**Phosphorus**	45 mg
Sodium	160 mg		

COOK'S TIP: White whole-wheat flour is available in the baking section of major supermarkets. The texture is similar to all-purpose flour, but has more fiber.

Peanut Butter and Banana Toasters

SERVES: 2 / **SERVING SIZE:** 1 piece of toast, 1 tablespoon peanut butter

1. Spread equal amounts of the peanut butter on each piece of toast, top with banana slices, and sprinkle evenly with the sugar substitute and cinnamon.

- 2 tablespoons low-sodium and 33% less sugar peanut butter
- 2 low-calorie 100% whole-wheat bread slices, toasted
- 3 tablespoons ripe banana slices
- ½ teaspoon pourable sugar substitute
- ¼ teaspoon ground cinnamon

EXCHANGES/CHOICES
1 starch, 1 fruit, 1 high-fat meat

Calories	150	**Potassium**	210 mg
Calories from Fat	70	**Total Carbohydrate**	15 g
Total Fat	8 g	Dietary Fiber	5 g
Saturated Fat	1.5 g	Sugars	4 g
Trans Fat	0 g	**Protein**	6 g
Cholesterol	0 mg	**Phosphorus**	95 mg
Sodium	150 mg		

Lemon-Strawberry Oatmeal

SERVES: 4 / **SERVING SIZE:** ⅓ cup oatmeal and ⅓ cup strawberry mixture

1⅓ cups sliced strawberries

2 teaspoons pourable sugar substitute

1 teaspoon grated lemon zest

1⅔ cups water, divided

⅔ cup quick-cooking oats

⅛ teaspoon salt

1 Stir together the strawberries, sugar substitute, lemon zest, and 2 tablespoons of the water. Set aside.

2 Bring the remaining 1½ cups water to a boil in a small saucepan, stir in the oats and salt, reduce heat to medium low, cover and cook 1 minute or until slightly thickened. Serve topped with strawberry mixture.

EXCHANGES/CHOICES
1 starch

Calories	80	**Potassium**	125 mg
Calories from Fat	10	**Total Carbohydrate**	15 g
Total Fat	1 g	Dietary Fiber	2 g
Saturated Fat	0 g	Sugars	4 g
Trans Fat	0 g	**Protein**	2 g
Cholesterol	0 mg	**Phosphorus**	65 mg
Sodium	55 mg		

Creamy Grits with Sauteed Chilies

SERVES: 4 / **SERVING SIZE:** ⅓ cup cooked grits and ¼ cup cooked peppers per serving

1 Heat the oil in a large nonstick skillet over medium-high heat. Cook the chilies 5 minutes or until just tender and beginning to brown, stirring frequently.

2 Meanwhile, bring the water to a boil in a small saucepan. Cook the grits according to package directions. Remove from heat.

3 Stir in the cream cheese until melted. Serve topped with equal amounts of the chilies.

- **1** teaspoon canola oil
- **3** medium poblano chili peppers, seeded and chopped
- **1½** cups water
- **⅓** cup quick cooking grits
- **2** ounces light herb and garlic cream cheese, such as Alouette

EXCHANGES/CHOICES
½ starch, 1 fat

Calories	90	**Potassium**	240 mg
Calories from Fat	45	**Total Carbohydrate**	15 g
Total Fat	4 g	Dietary Fiber	0 g
Saturated Fat	1.5 g	Sugars	1 g
Trans Fat	0 g	**Protein**	3 g
Cholesterol	10 mg	**Phosphorus**	25 mg
Sodium	120 mg		

Tomato, Bacon, and Cheddar Grits, PAGE 29

Tomato, Bacon, and Cheddar Grits

SERVES: 4 / **SERVING SIZE:** ⅓ cup cooked grits and about ⅓ cup vegetable mixture

1 Heat a large nonstick skillet over medium-high heat. Cook the bacon 5 minutes or until crisp, turning occasionally. Drain bacon on paper towels. Discard bacon grease, return skillet to medium-high heat, add the peppers and ¼ cup of the water to the skillet, and cook 5 minutes or until water has evaporated and peppers are tender-crisp. Stir in the tomatoes, onion, thyme, and hot sauce. Cook 2 minutes or until tomatoes are just tender. Remove from heat.

2 Meanwhile, bring the remaining 1½ cups water to a boil in a small saucepan. Cook the grits according to package directions. Remove from heat.

3 Serve grits topped with vegetable mixture and cheese and crumble the bacon over all.

8	center-cut turkey bacon slices
1	cup diced green bell pepper
1¾	cups water, divided use
1	cup grape tomatoes, quartered
½	cup finely chopped green onion (green and white parts total)
¼	teaspoon dried thyme leaves
2	teaspoons mild Louisiana hot sauce (or to taste), such as Frank's
⅓	cup quick-cooking grits
1	ounce shredded reduced-fat sharp cheddar cheese

COOK'S TIP: For additional protein, scramble and cook 1 cup egg substitute, top the grits with the eggs, and spoon the vegetables, cheese, and bacon on top.

EXCHANGES/CHOICES
½ starch, 1 high-fat meat

Calories	140	**Potassium**	310 mg
Calories from Fat	70	**Total Carbohydrate**	15 g
Total Fat	8 g	Dietary Fiber	2 g
Saturated Fat	2.5 g	Sugars	2 g
Trans Fat	0 g	**Protein**	10 g
Cholesterol	25 mg	**Phosphorus**	170 mg
Sodium	630 mg		

Buttery Orange and Hot Apple Slices

SERVES: 4 / **SERVING SIZE:** ½ cup

3 cups red apple slices, such as Gala (about 2 medium apples total)

2 tablespoons diet margarine

2 tablespoons sugar-free orange marmalade

¼ teaspoon almond extract or

½ teaspoon vanilla

1 Place the apples and diet margarine in a shallow microwave-safe pan, such as a glass pie pan. Cover and cook on high setting for 5 minutes or until just tender-crisp, and stir in the marmalade and almond extract until apples are well coated. Serve hot or at room temperature.

EXCHANGES/CHOICES
1 fruit, ½ fat

Calories	75	**Potassium**	90 mg
Calories from Fat	30	**Total Carbohydrate**	14 g
Total Fat	3 g	Dietary Fiber	2 g
Saturated Fat	1 g	Sugars	9 g
Trans Fat	0 g	**Protein**	0 g
Cholesterol	0 mg	**Phosphorus**	9 mg
Sodium	40 mg		

COOK'S TIP: Use as a breakfast side to turkey sausage or Canadian bacon. Or serve as a side to an entrée such as pork or chicken.

Raspberry Lemon Honeydew

SERVES: 4 / **SERVING SIZE:** ½ cup

 1 Place the honeydew in a shallow serving bowl or rimmed plate.

 2 Whisk together the jam, lemon zest, and juice. Spoon evenly over the fruit. Sprinkle with the mint, if desired.

2	cups honeydew cubes, about ¾-inch pieces
2	tablespoons sugar-free raspberry jam
1–2	teaspoons grated lemon zest
2–3	tablespoons lemon juice
2	tablespoons finely chopped fresh mint (optional)

FOR VARIATION: Substitute for honeydew with 3 cups diced watermelon and 1 medium kiwi, peeled and diced

EXCHANGES/CHOICES
1 fruit

Calories	50	**Potassium**	320 mg
Calories from Fat	0	**Total Carbohydrate**	15 g
Total Fat	0 g	Dietary Fiber	1 g
Saturated Fat	0 g	Sugars	9 g
Trans Fat	0 g	**Protein**	1 g
Cholesterol	0 mg	**Phosphorus**	15 mg
Sodium	15 mg		

Yogurt with Syrup'd Strawberries and Almonds

SERVES: 4 / **SERVING SIZE:** ½ cup yogurt, about ⅓ cup strawberry mixture, and 2 teaspoons almonds

1⅓ cups sliced strawberries
½ cup water
2 tablespoons plus 2 teaspoons pourable sugar substitute
½ teaspoon almond extract
2 cups nonfat, plain Greek yogurt
2 tablespoons plus 2 teaspoons sliced almonds, coarsely crumbled

1. In a medium bowl, combine the strawberries, water, sugar substitute, and extract. Mash slightly with a fork and, if time allows, let stand 15 minutes at room temperature.

2. Spoon equal amounts of the yogurt in each of 4 dessert dishes or small bowls. Spoon equal amounts of the strawberry mixture (about ½ cup) on top of each serving and sprinkle with the almonds.

EXCHANGES/CHOICES
1 milk, ½ medium-fat meat

Calories	110	**Potassium**	260 mg
Calories from Fat	20	**Total Carbohydrate**	15 g
Total Fat	2 g	Dietary Fiber	2 g
Saturated Fat	0 g	Sugars	6 g
Trans Fat	0 g	**Protein**	13 g
Cholesterol	5 mg	**Phosphorus**	180 mg
Sodium	40 mg		

Citrus Blueberry Yogurt Bowls

SERVES: 4 / **SERVING SIZE:** ½ cup yogurt and 3 tablespoons blueberry mixture

1 Whisk together the preserves, sugar substitute, and zest in a small bowl. Gently stir in the blueberries until well coated.

2 Spoon ½ cup yogurt into each of 4 bowls and spoon the berry mixture on top.

- **2** tablespoons sugar-free raspberry preserves
- **1** teaspoon pourable sugar substitute
- **½** teaspoon grated lemon zest or orange zest
- **¾** cup fresh or frozen, thawed blueberries
- **2** cups nonfat, plain Greek yogurt

EXCHANGES/CHOICES
½ carbohydrate, ½ skim milk

Calories	100	**Potassium**	180 mg
Calories from Fat	0	**Total Carbohydrate**	15 g
Total Fat	0.5 g	Dietary Fiber	1 g
Saturated Fat	0 g	Sugars	11 g
Trans Fat	0 g	**Protein**	11 g
Cholesterol	0 mg	**Phosphorus**	160 mg
Sodium	45 mg		

Quiche in a Cup

SERVES: 1 / **SERVING SIZE:** 1 cup

⅓ cup frozen corn, thawed

1 ounce Canadian bacon, diced

¼ cup diced green bell pepper or green onion

¼ cup egg substitute

1 tablespoon shredded reduced-fat cheddar cheese

1. Coat a 6-ounce ramekin with cooking spray. Place the corn, Canadian bacon, and bell peppper in the ramekin, stir and pour the egg substitute over all and top with the cheese. Cover with plastic wrap and microwave on high for 3 minutes or until puffed and egg is just set.

2. Let stand 2–3 minutes, if time allows, to absorb flavors and cool slightly.

EXCHANGES/CHOICES
1 starch, 2 lean meat

Calories	170	**Potassium**	420 mg
Calories from Fat	45	**Total Carbohydrate**	15 g
Total Fat	5 g	Dietary Fiber	2 g
Saturated Fat	2.5 g	Sugars	4 g
Trans Fat	0 g	**Protein**	18 g
Cholesterol	20 mg	**Phosphorus**	240 mg
Sodium	480 mg		

Ham and Potato Skillet Quiche

SERVES: 4 / **SERVING SIZE:** ¼ quiche

1. Heat the oil in a medium nonstick skillet over medium-high heat. Add the onions and bell pepper and cook 5 minutes or until onions are tender, stirring occasionally.

2. Meanwhile, in a medium bowl, whisk together the eggs, egg whites, milk, and parsley until well blended. Stir in the potatoes and ham.

3. Reduce the heat to medium low, pour potato mixture evenly over all, cover, and cook 16–17 minutes or until eggs are set and knife inserted in center comes out clean. Remove from heat, sprinkle evenly with the salt, and top with the cheese. Let stand 10 minutes to absorb flavors and allow cheese to melt. Cut into four wedges to serve.

1	tablespoon canola oil
1	cup diced onion
1	cup diced red bell pepper
2	large eggs
2	large egg whites
¼	cup fat-free milk
¼	cup chopped fresh parsley
2	cups frozen, thawed country-style hash brown potatoes
4	ounces extra-lean diced ham
⅛	teaspoon salt
1	ounce shredded reduced-fat sharp cheddar

EXCHANGES/CHOICES
½ starch, 1 vegetable, 2 lean meat, 1 fat

Calories	190	**Potassium**	560 mg
Calories from Fat	80	**Total Carbohydrate**	15 g
Total Fat	9 g	Dietary Fiber	2 g
Saturated Fat	2.5 g	Sugars	4 g
Trans Fat	0 g	**Protein**	14 g
Cholesterol	120 mg	**Phosphorus**	260 mg
Sodium	570 mg		

Baked Spinach-Bacon Casserole

SERVES: 6 / **SERVING SIZE:** 1 cup

6 bacon slices, chopped
1 tablespoon extra-virgin olive oil
1 cup diced onion
1 (10-ounce) package frozen chopped spinach, thawed and squeezed dry
2 cups egg substitute
½ cup fat-free milk
½ cup fat-free plain Greek yogurt
¼ teaspoon salt, divided use
⅛ teaspoon cayenne (optional)
2 ounces reduced-fat thin, sliced Swiss cheese, torn in small pieces
½ cup panko bread crumbs
5 ounces grape tomatoes, quartered

1 Preheat oven to 325°F.

2 Cook bacon in a medium skillet over medium-high heat until crisp. Drain on paper towels. Discard bacon grease and paper towel. Dry skillet. Return skillet to medium heat, heat 1 teaspoon of the olive oil, and cook onion 4 minutes or until tender. Remove from heat. Add to a medium bowl with the spinach, egg substitute, milk, yogurt, ⅛ teaspoon salt, and cayenne. Stir until well blended.

3 Pour the spinach mixture into an 11 × 7-inch baking dish coated with cooking spray. Bake 30 minutes, sprinkle with the cheese, breadcrumbs, bacon, and top with tomatoes, drizzle the remaining 2 teaspoons oil evenly over all, and cook 5 minutes or until knife inserted comes out clean. Sprinkle with remaining salt and let stand 10 minutes.

EXCHANGES/CHOICES

½ starch, 2 vegetable, 2 medium-fat meat

Calories	230	**Potassium**	670 mg
Calories from Fat	90	**Total Carbohydrate**	15 g
Total Fat	10 g	Dietary Fiber	3 g
Saturated Fat	2.5 g	Sugars	5 g
Trans Fat	0 g	**Protein**	22 g
Cholesterol	15 mg	**Phosphorus**	300 mg
Sodium	500 mg		

Lemon Asparagus Panko Frittata

SERVES: 4 / **SERVING SIZE:** ¼ frittata

1 Heat oil in medium nonstick skillet over medium-high heat. Tilt skillet to coat bottom lightly. Cook the breadcrumbs 2–3 minutes or until golden, stirring constantly. Remove from heat, stir in the lemon zest and ¼ teaspoon salt and set aside on separate plate.

2 Whisk together the eggs, egg white, milk, onion, dill, black pepper, and ¼ teaspoon salt. Set aside.

3 Combine asparagus and water in the skillet. Bring to a boil over medium-high heat, reduce heat to medium low, cover, and cook 2–3 minutes or until asparagus is just tender-crisp. Drain in a colander, shaking off excess liquid.

4 Return asparagus to the skillet over medium-low heat. Pour the egg mixture evenly over all, cover, and cook 12–13 minutes or until eggs are almost set. Remove from the heat, sprinkle with the breadcrumb mixture, and let stand 10–15 minutes, uncovered, to allow frittata to firm slightly and absorb flavors.

5 Run a rubber spatula around edge and under frittata to loosen from pan. Slide frittata onto a plate or cutting board. Cut into 4 wedges.

2	teaspoons canola oil
1	cup panko breadcrumbs
2	tablespoons grated lemon zest
½	teaspoon salt, divided use
5	large eggs, lightly beaten
1	egg white, lightly beaten
¼	cup fat-free milk
⅓	cup finely chopped green onion
2	tablespoons chopped fresh dill
¼	teaspoon black pepper
6	ounces asparagus, trimmed and cut into 2-inch pieces
¼	cup water

EXCHANGES/CHOICES
½ starch, 2 vegetable, 1 medium-fat meat, ½ fat

Calories	190	**Potassium**	270 mg
Calories from Fat	80	**Total Carbohydrate**	15 g
Total Fat	9 g	Dietary Fiber	2 g
Saturated Fat	2.5 g	Sugars	3 g
Trans Fat	0 g	**Protein**	12 g
Cholesterol	230 mg	**Phosphorus**	190 mg
Sodium	420 mg		

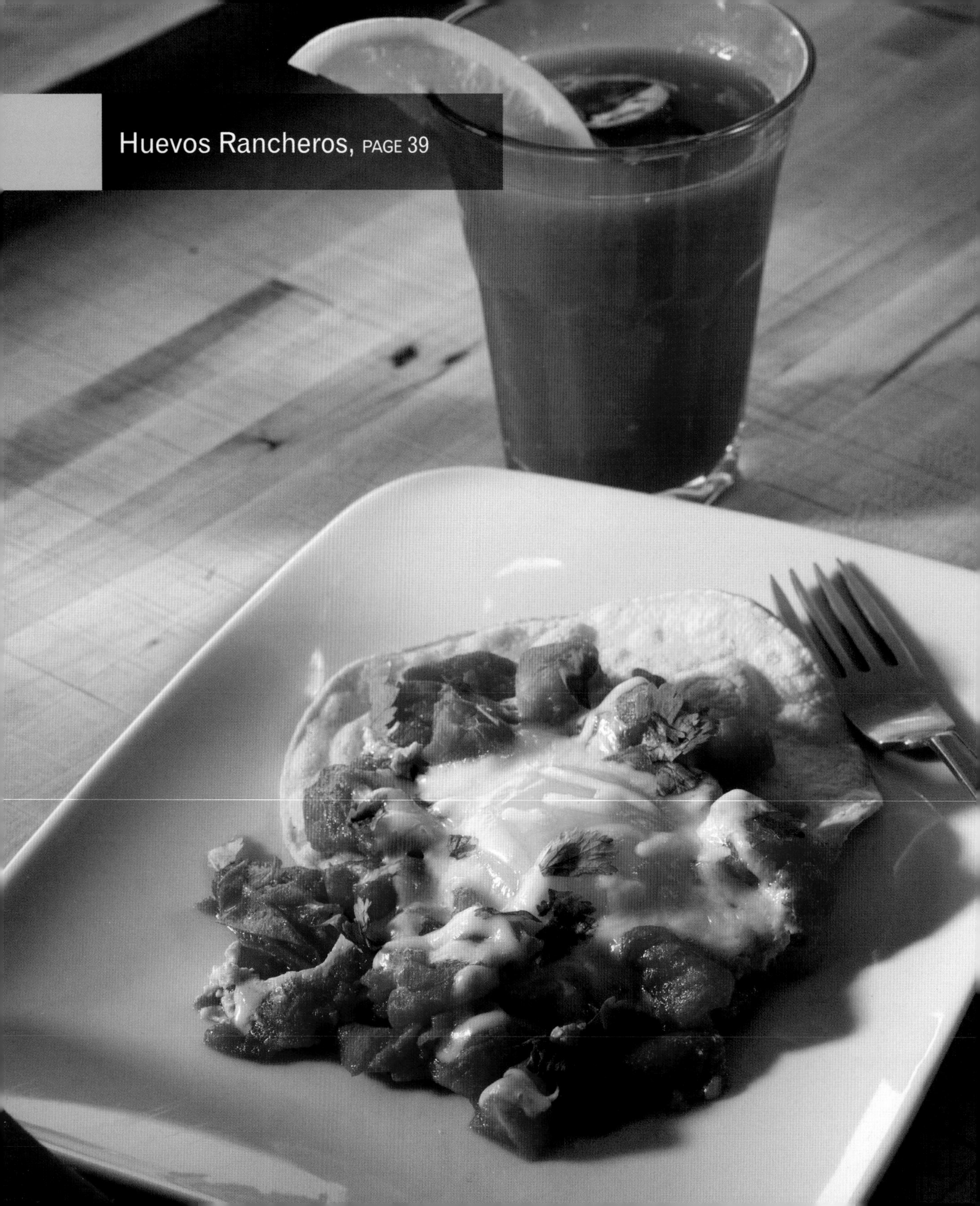

Huevos Rancheros, PAGE 39

Huevos Rancheros

SERVES: 4 / **SERVING SIZE:** 1 stack

1 Preheat oven to 425°F.

2 Place tortillas on baking sheet and bake 3 minutes on each side.

3 Meanwhile, place the tomatoes, cumin, cayenne, and salt in a medium nonstick skillet and bring to a boil over medium-high heat. Reduce heat to medium low and cook, covered, 3 minutes or until slightly thickened. Break one egg into a measuring cup. Carefully slide egg onto the tomato mixture. Repeat with the remaining eggs. Simmer gently over medium heat, covered, 2½ to 3 minutes or until whites are completely set and yolks just begin to thicken slightly.

4 Place a tortilla on each of four dinner plates. Top with the tomato mixture and eggs. Sprinkle with cheese and cilantro.

4 corn tortillas
1 (14.5-ounce) can no-salt-added diced tomatoes, drained
1 teaspoon ground cumin
⅛ teaspoon cayenne pepper (optional)
½ teaspoon salt
4 large eggs
1 ounce shredded part-skim mozzarella cheese or reduced-fat feta
¼ cup chopped cilantro

EXCHANGES/CHOICES
1 starch, 1 lean meat, 1 fat

Calories	160	**Potassium**	380 mg
Calories from Fat	60	**Total Carbohydrate**	15 g
Total Fat	7 g	Dietary Fiber	3 g
Saturated Fat	2.5 g	Sugars	3 g
Trans Fat	0 g	**Protein**	10 g
Cholesterol	190 mg	**Phosphorus**	240 mg
Sodium	330 mg		

Poached Eggs on Chopped Toast

SERVES: 4 / **SERVING SIZE:** 1 poached egg and 1½ slices of toast per serving

8	cups water
4	large eggs
¼	teaspoon salt
	Black pepper to taste
6	slices reduced-calorie whole-wheat bread
2	tablespoons diet margarine

1 Pour water into a large nonstick skillet and bring to a boil over medium-high heat. Reduce heat and simmer. Break 1 egg into a measuring cup. Carefully slide egg into simmering water, holding the lip of the cup as close to the water as possible. Repeat with remaining eggs, allowing each egg an equal amount of space.

2 Simmer eggs, uncovered, for 3–5 minutes or until the whites are completely set and yolks begin to thicken slightly. Remove eggs with a slotted spoon. Sprinkle with salt and pepper.

3 Meanwhile, toast the bread slices, spread the diet margarine evenly over slices, and cut into bite-size pieces. Place chopped bread in four shallow soup bowls and top each serving with a poached egg. Sprinkle with salt and pepper.

EXCHANGES/CHOICES
1 starch, 1 medium-fat meat, 1 fat

Calories	190	**Potassium**	170 mg
Calories from Fat	80	**Total Carbohydrate**	15 g
Total Fat	9 g	Dietary Fiber	3 g
Saturated Fat	2.5 g	Sugars	2 g
Trans Fat	0 g	**Protein**	11 g
Cholesterol	190 mg	**Phosphorus**	175 mg
Sodium	380 mg		

Creamed Eggs on Toast

SERVES: 4 / **SERVING SIZE:** 1 toast slice, about ½ cup sliced egg, and ¼ cup sauce

1 In a small bowl, whisk together ½ cup of the milk and the cornstarch until cornstarch is dissolved. Pour mixture into a medium saucepan and add the remaining milk. Bring just to a boil over medium-high heat, stirring frequently. Continue to boil 1 full minute, stirring constantly.

2 Remove from heat and stir in the margarine and salt.

3 Arrange a toast slice on each dinner plate. Slice or chop the eggs and top the toast slices with equal amounts of the eggs. Spoon the sauce over each serving and sprinkle with the black pepper.

1 cup fat-free milk, divided use
1 tablespoon cornstarch
2 tablespoons diet margarine
¼ teaspoon salt
4 reduced-calorie whole-wheat bread slices, toasted
7 hardboiled eggs, peeled (discard 2 yolks)
   Black pepper to taste

EXCHANGES/CHOICES
1 starch, 1½ medium-fat meat

Calories	190	**Potassium**	230 mg
Calories from Fat	70	**Total Carbohydrate**	15 g
Total Fat	8 g	Dietary Fiber	3 g
Saturated Fat	2.5 g	Sugars	5 g
Trans Fat	0 g	**Protein**	14 g
Cholesterol	190 mg	**Phosphorus**	185 mg
Sodium	340 mg		

Open-Faced Egg Sandwiches

SERVES: 4 / **SERVING SIZE:** 1 sandwich

4 reduced-calorie whole-wheat bread slices

1 tablespoon plus 1 teaspoon diet margarine

2 teaspoons Dijon mustard

2 medium tomatoes, cut into 8 slices

2 cups arugula

1 teaspoon canola oil

2 cups fat-free egg substitute

2 ounces shredded reduced-fat sharp cheddar cheese

1 Preheat broiler.

2 Place the bread slices on a baking sheet and broil 1½ minutes on each side or until lightly toasted, watching closely not to burn. Remove from broiler and set aside. Do not turn off broiler.

3 Stir together the diet margarine and mustard in a small bowl until well blended. Spread equal amounts on top of each piece of toast. Place the bread slices on the baking sheet. Top each with equal amounts of the tomato slices and top with the arugula and set aside.

4 Heat the oil in a medium nonstick skillet over medium heat. Cook the egg substitute for 2 minutes, stirring occasionally. Spoon equal amounts of the egg on top of the arugula and sprinkle evenly with the cheese. Run under the broiler 1–2 minutes or until the cheese is melted.

EXCHANGES/CHOICES
½ starch, 1 vegetable, 2½ lean meat

Calories	190	**Potassium**	420 mg
Calories from Fat	50	**Total Carbohydrate**	15 g
Total Fat	6 g	Dietary Fiber	4 g
Saturated Fat	2.5 g	Sugars	4 g
Trans Fat	0 g	**Protein**	20 g
Cholesterol	10 mg	**Phosphorus**	140 mg
Sodium	500 mg		

Skillet Chicken Sausage with Potatoes

SERVES: 4 / **SERVING SIZE:** 1 cup

1. Heat 1 teaspoon of the oil in a large non-stick skillet over medium-high heat. Cook the sausage 5 minutes or until lightly browned, stirring frequently and set aside. Add the remaining 2 teaspoons oil to the skillet. Cook the peppers 4 minutes or until beginning to richly brown. Add the remaining ingredients, reduce the heat to medium low, cover, and cook 7 minutes or until mushrooms are tender.

1 tablespoon canola oil, divided use

8 ounces chicken apple sausage, thinly sliced

¾ cup thinly sliced red bell pepper

4 ounces whole mushrooms, quartered

1 (14.5-ounce) can diced or sliced potatoes, rinsed and drained

½ cup chopped green onion

COOK'S TIP: To make this quick dish even quicker, buy pre-sliced mushrooms and bell peppers and pre-chopped green onions in the produce section of major supermarkets.

EXCHANGES/CHOICES
1 starch, 1 vegetable, 2 lean meats

Calories	210	**Potassium**	370 mg
Calories from Fat	110	**Total Carbohydrate**	15 g
Total Fat	12 g	Dietary Fiber	3 g
Saturated Fat	2.5 g	Sugars	3 g
Trans Fat	0 g	**Protein**	10 g
Cholesterol	55 mg	**Phosphorus**	140 mg
Sodium	590 mg		

Strawberry Power Juicer or Slush

SERVES: 5 / **SERVING SIZE:** ⅔ cup

3	cups frozen unsweetened strawberries
1	cup shredded kale
½	cup apple juice
½	cup water
3	tablespoons pourable sugar substitute
2	tablespoons lemon juice
½	teaspoon almond extract

 Combine all ingredients in a blender and purée until smooth.

EXCHANGES/CHOICES

½ fruit, 1 vegetable

Calories	65	**Potassium**	270 mg
Calories from Fat	0	**Total Carbohydrate**	15 g
Total Fat	0 g	Dietary Fiber	3 g
Saturated Fat	0 g	Sugars	7 g
Trans Fat	0 g	**Protein**	1 g
Cholesterol	0 mg	**Phosphorus**	30 mg
Sodium	10 mg		

Mighty Tomato Juice

SERVES: 2 / **SERVING SIZE:** 1¼ cup

 Combine all ingredients in a blender and purée until smooth.

2	cups low-sodium tomato juice
4	ounces diced pimiento
½	(4-ounce) can chopped mild green chilies or ¼ cup picante sauce
¼–⅓	cup chopped cilantro
½	medium jalapeño, seeded
2	tablespoons lemon juice

EXCHANGES/CHOICES
3 vegetable

Calories	70	**Potassium**	570 mg
Calories from Fat	5	**Total Carbohydrate**	15 g
Total Fat	0.5 g	Dietary Fiber	3 g
Saturated Fat	0 g	Sugars	9 g
Trans Fat	0 g	**Protein**	2 g
Cholesterol	0 mg	**Phosphorus**	50 mg
Sodium	390 mg		

Purple Swirl Smoothie

SERVES: 2 / **SERVING SIZE:** ¾ cup

¾ cup nonfat plain Greek yogurt
⅔ cup fresh or frozen blueberries
2 tablespoons pourable sugar substitute
1½ teaspoons vanilla extract
1 cup ice cubes

1 Place all ingredients in a blender and purée until smooth.

EXCHANGES/CHOICES
1 fruit, ½ carbohydrate, 1 lean meat

Calories	90	**Potassium**	160 mg
Calories from Fat	5	**Total Carbohydrate**	12 g
Total Fat	0.5 g	Dietary Fiber	1 g
Saturated Fat	0 g	Sugars	12 g
Trans Fat	0 g	**Protein**	9 g
Cholesterol	<5 mg	**Phosphorus**	120 mg
Sodium	30 mg		

Creamy Peanutty Chiller

SERVES: 2 / **SERVING SIZE:** 1 cup

1 Place all ingredients in a blender and purée until smooth.

1 cup fat-free milk
4 teaspoons low-sodium and 33% less sugar peanut butter
¼ cup sliced bananas
1½ tablespoons pourable sugar substitute
½ teaspoon vanilla extract or more
1 cup ice cubes

EXCHANGES/CHOICES
½ skim milk, ½ carbohydrate, 1 high-fat meat

Calories	130	**Potassium**	330 mg
Calories from Fat	50	**Total Carbohydrate**	15 g
Total Fat	6 g	Dietary Fiber	1 g
Saturated Fat	1 g	Sugars	12 g
Trans Fat	0 g	**Protein**	7 g
Cholesterol	<5 mg	**Phosphorus**	170 mg
Sodium	50 mg		

Lunch

SANDWICHES AND MORE

Knife and Fork Beefy Corn Tortilla Piles

Bacon, Lettuce, and Pepper Tortilla Wraps

Picante Quesadilla Wedges

Curried Tuna and Sweet Pepper
  Open-Face Sandwich

Ham-Swiss on Rye with Creamy
  Coleslaw Topping

Italian Sausage Bread Shells

Chicken and Blue Cheese Pita Pockets

Deviled Egg Salad Pitas

Long Leaf Chicken-Avocado Wraps

Protein Hummus and Crisp Veggies

SOUPS

Creamy Chicken Corn Soup

Chicken, Pasta and Spinach Soup

Sausage, Bean, and Carrot Soup

Tomato-Cilantro Soup

Black Bean–Green Pepper Soup

MAIN SALADS

Asian Chicken, Cabbage, and Cilantro Salad

Layered Chicken Taco Salad

Chicken and Toasted Pecan Salad

Asian Chicken–Wild Rice Salad

Turkey and Swiss Stuffed Eggs

Turkey, Greens, and Strawberry Almond Salad

Chunky Veggie Egg and Bean Salad

Garbanzo-Feta Salad

Grilled Sirloin and Blue Cheese Salad

Ham and Edamame Chop Salad

Knife and Fork Beefy Corn Tortilla Piles

SERVES: 4 / **SERVING SIZE:** ¼ recipe

1	teaspoon canola oil
12	ounces extra-lean ground beef
¾	cup diced tomatoes, divided use
2	teaspoons ground cumin
½	teaspoon salt
⅛	teaspoon cayenne (optional)
4	(6-inch) corn tortillas
¼	cup chopped fresh cilantro
2	cups shredded romaine lettuce
1	ounce shredded low-fat sharp cheddar cheese
1	medium lime, cut in 4 wedges

1 Heat the oil in a large nonstick skillet over medium-high heat. Brown beef, stir in ½ cup of the tomatoes, cumin, salt, and cayenne and cook 1 minute or until tomatoes are soft, stirring frequently.

2 Warm tortillas according to package directions. Place one on each of 4 dinner plates. Spoon equal amounts of the beef mixture on top of each tortilla. Sprinkle evenly with the cilantro, lettuce, remaining tomatoes, and cheese. Squeeze the lime juice evenly over all.

EXCHANGES/CHOICES
1 starch, 3 lean meat

Calories	210	**Potassium**	520 mg
Calories from Fat	60	**Total Carbohydrate**	15 g
Total Fat	7 g	Dietary Fiber	3 g
Saturated Fat	2.5 g	Sugars	2 g
Trans Fat	0 g	**Protein**	22 g
Cholesterol	55 mg	**Phosphorus**	300 mg
Sodium	320 mg		

Bacon, Lettuce, and Pepper Tortilla Wraps

SERVES: 4 / **SERVING SIZE:** 2 slices bacon, 1 tablespoon spread, and about 1 cup vegetables

 1 Heat the tortillas according to package microwave directions.

2 In a small bowl, stir together the mayonnaise, sour cream and paprika. Spread equal amounts down the center of each tortilla. Top with equal amounts of the bacon, lettuce, bell pepper, and onion. Fold two sides together, overlapping slightly.

- **4** low-carb, high-fiber flour tortillas
- **2** tablespoons light mayonnaise
- **2** tablespoons fat-free sour cream
- **½** teaspoon smoked paprika or chipotle powder
- **8** slices center-cut low-sodium turkey bacon, cooked
- **4** cups shredded Romaine lettuce
- **½** cup diced green bell pepper or poblano
- **¼** cup finely chopped green onion, (green and white parts total)

EXCHANGES/CHOICES
1 starch, 2 lean meat, ½ fat

Calories	180	**Potassium**	200 mg
Calories from Fat	80	**Total Carbohydrate**	15 g
Total Fat	9 g	Dietary Fiber	9 g
Saturated Fat	2 g	Sugars	1 g
Trans Fat	0 g	**Protein**	14 g
Cholesterol	40 mg	**Phosphorus**	30 mg
Sodium	580 mg		

Picante Quesadilla Wedges

SERVES: 4 / **SERVING SIZE:** 3 wedges

3	ounces part-skim low-fat mozzarella cheese, shredded
½	cup canned no-salt-added black beans, rinsed and drained
½	cup picante sauce
¼	cup chopped cilantro
½	teaspoon ground cumin
3	low-carb, high-fiber flour tortillas, such as La Tortilla Factory, cut into 4 wedges
1½	teaspoons canola oil
¼	cup fat-free sour cream

1 Combine the cheese, beans, picante sauce, cilantro, and cumin in a medium bowl. Spoon equal amounts of the bean mixture on one half of each tortilla wedge.

2 Fold over tortillas and press down gently to allow them to adhere.

3 Heat the oil in a large nonstick skillet over medium heat. Tilt the skillet to lightly coat bottom. Cook tortillas 2 minutes on each side or until cheese has melted and tortillas are golden.

EXCHANGES/CHOICES
1 starch, 1 lean meat, 1 fat

Calories	150	**Potassium**	220 mg
Calories from Fat	70	**Total Carbohydrate**	15 g
Total Fat	8 g	Dietary Fiber	8 g
Saturated Fat	2.5 g	Sugars	1 g
Trans Fat	0 g	**Protein**	11 g
Cholesterol	10 mg	**Phosphorus**	140 mg
Sodium	550 mg		

Curried Tuna and Sweet Pepper Open-Face Sandwich

SERVES: 4 / **SERVING SIZE:** 1 cup tuna mixture and 1 slice toast

1 Place tuna in a colander, rinse under water, and drain well by pressing with a rubber spatula to release excess liquid.

2 In a medium bowl, combine the drained tuna, eggs, mayonnaise, sugar substitute, and curry powder. Stir until well blended. Stir in the celery and bell pepper. Serve equal amounts over the toasted bread.

2	(5-ounce) cans tuna in water
2	large hardboiled eggs, peeled and finely chopped
1/3	cup light mayonnaise
1	tablespoon pourable sugar substitute
1–1½	teaspoons curry powder
1	cup diced celery
1	cup finely chopped red bell pepper
4	slices reduced-calorie whole-wheat bread, toasted

EXCHANGES/CHOICES
1 starch, 3 lean meat, 1 fat

Calories	250	**Potassium**	400 mg
Calories from Fat	90	**Total Carbohydrate**	15 g
Total Fat	10 g	Dietary Fiber	4 g
Saturated Fat	2.5 g	Sugars	4 g
Trans Fat	0 g	**Protein**	24 g
Cholesterol	130 mg	**Phosphorus**	250 mg
Sodium	550 mg		

Ham-Swiss on Rye with Creamy Coleslaw Topping

SERVES: 4 / **SERVING SIZE:** 1 open-faced sandwich and ½ cup cabbage mixture

4	slices reduced-calorie rye bread with caraway
4	ounces thinly sliced extra-lean ham
2	ounces very thinly sliced Swiss cheese
1	medium jalapeño, cut into thin slices (not seeded)
1	tablespoon water
4	teaspoons light mayonnaise
1	teaspoon prepared mustard
1	teaspoon dried dill weed
½	teaspoon pourable sugar substitute
2	cups finely shredded cabbage

1. Top each of the bread slices with equal amounts of the ham and cheese and arrange the jalapeño slices evenly over all. Place 2 of the bread slices on a microwave-safe plate and microwave on high for 1–2 minutes or until the cheese has melted. Repeat with the remaining two bread slices.

2. Meanwhile, in a medium bowl, whisk together the water, mayonnaise, mustard, dill, and sugar substitute. Add the cabbage and toss until well coated. Top each bread slice with equal amounts of the cabbage mixture.

EXCHANGES/CHOICES

½ starch, 1 vegetable, 1½ lean meat

Calories	130	**Potassium**	300 mg
Calories from Fat	30	**Total Carbohydrate**	13 g
Total Fat	3 g	Dietary Fiber	3 g
Saturated Fat	1 g	Sugars	3 g
Trans Fat	0 g	**Protein**	12 g
Cholesterol	20 mg	**Phosphorus**	200 mg
Sodium	510 mg		

Italian Sausage Bread Shells

SERVES: 4 / **SERVING SIZE:** ⅓ cup filling and 1 bread shell

1 Cut each piece of bread in half crosswise. Hollow out top and bottom halves of bread, leaving a ½-inch-thick shell; discard torn bread.

2 Set oven to 350°F. (No need to preheat oven.) Place the bread "shells" on a cookie sheet and bake 4–5 minutes or until bottoms are lightly browned. Remove from heat and let stand 1–2 minutes to harden slightly.

3 Meanwhile, heat the oil in a medium non-stick skillet over medium-high heat. Cook the sausage 3 minutes or until browned, breaking up larger pieces while cooking. Remove from heat, stir in the tomatoes and basil. Gently stir in the feta. Spoon equal amounts into each bread shell.

6 ounces Italian bread, cut in half lengthwise
1 teaspoon canola oil
4 ounces hot or mild Italian turkey sausage, casings removed
1 medium plum tomato, finely chopped
¼ cup chopped fresh basil
1 ounce reduced-fat feta, crumbled

EXCHANGES/CHOICES
1 starch, 1 medium-fat meat

Calories	150	**Potassium**	170 mg
Calories from Fat	50	**Total Carbohydrate**	15 g
Total Fat	5 g	Dietary Fiber	1 g
Saturated Fat	2 g	Sugars	2 g
Trans Fat	0 g	**Protein**	8 g
Cholesterol	20 mg	**Phosphorus**	110 mg
Sodium	500 mg		

Chicken and Blue Cheese Pita Pockets

SERVES: 4 / **SERVING SIZE:** 1 cup romaine mixture and 1 pita half

2	cups shredded Romaine lettuce
1⅓	cups cooked diced chicken breast
¼	cup finely chopped red onion
1½	ounces reduced-fat blue cheese crumbles
2	tablespoons capers, drained
1½	tablespoons extra-virgin olive oil
2	teaspoons lemon juice
½	teaspoon dried oregano leaves
2	whole-wheat pita rounds, cut in half crosswise (forming 4 pockets or half moons)

1 In a medium bowl, combine all ingredients, except the pita halves. Warm pitas according to package directions.

2 Toss the romaine mixture until well blended and fill each pita half with equal amounts of the mixture.

EXCHANGES/CHOICES
1 starch, 1 vegetable, 2½ lean meat, 1 fat

Calories	250	**Potassium**	270 mg
Calories from Fat	90	**Total Carbohydrate**	15 g
Total Fat	10 g	Dietary Fiber	3 g
Saturated Fat	2.5 g	Sugars	1 g
Trans Fat	0 g	**Protein**	21 g
Cholesterol	45 mg	**Phosphorus**	200 mg
Sodium	440 mg		

Deviled Egg Salad Pitas

SERVES: 4 / **SERVING SIZE:** 1 pita half, ½ cup lettuce, and ½ cup egg mixture

1 Chop the eggs and place in a medium bowl with the mayonnaise, vinegar, mustard, and salt. Stir until well blended. Stir in the peppers.

2 Warm pita halves according to package directions. Place ½ cup lettuce in each pita, and spoon equal amounts of the egg mixture on top of the lettuce. Sprinkle with black pepper.

5	large hard-boiled eggs, peeled, discarding 1 yolk
2	tablespoons light mayonnaise
2	teaspoons cider vinegar
½	teaspoon prepared mustard
¼	teaspoon salt
⅓	cup finely chopped green bell pepper
2	cups shredded Romaine lettuce
2	whole-wheat pita rounds, halved, warmed
	Black pepper to taste

EXCHANGES/CHOICES
1 starch, 1 vegetable, 1 medium-fat meat

Calories	170	**Potassium**	210 mg
Calories from Fat	70	**Total Carbohydrate**	15 g
Total Fat	8 g	Dietary Fiber	2 g
Saturated Fat	1.5 g	Sugars	1 g
Trans Fat	0 g	**Protein**	10 g
Cholesterol	215 mg	**Phosphorus**	155 mg
Sodium	420 mg		

Long Leaf Chicken-Avocado Wraps, PAGE 59

Long Leaf Chicken-Avocado Wraps

SERVES: 4 / **SERVING SIZE:** 2 lettuce wraps

1 Season the chicken with the paprika. Coat a medium skillet with cooking spray and place over medium heat until hot. Cook chicken 5 minutes on each side or until no longer pink in center. Place on cutting board and thinly slice.

2 In a small bowl, mix together the avocado, sour cream, and garlic. Spread equal amounts on each Romaine leaf. Top with equal amounts of the picante sauce, chicken, cilantro, olives and cheese. Fold long sides together to resemble a hot dog bun. Serve with lime wedges.

3	(4-ounce) boneless, skinless chicken breasts, rinsed and patted dry
1½	teaspoons smoked paprika or chili powder
	Cooking spray
1	ripe avocado, peeled and mashed with a fork
½	cup fat-free sour cream
1	medium garlic clove, minced
8	large Romaine lettuce leaves
½	cup chipotle or regular picante sauce
½	cup chopped fresh cilantro
16	pitted ripe olives, sliced
1	oz shredded reduced-fat sharp cheddar cheese
1	medium lime, quartered

COOK'S TIP: This makes a great "portable" lunch or a fun snack. Make them up in individual servings in "to go" plastic containers and refrigerate until you're ready to go!

EXCHANGES/CHOICES
½ starch, 2 vegetables, 2½ lean meat, 1 fat

Calories	240	**Potassium**	700 mg
Calories from Fat	100	**Total Carbohydrate**	14 g
Total Fat	11 g	Dietary Fiber	4 g
Saturated Fat	2.5 g	Sugars	1 g
Trans Fat	0 g	**Protein**	23 g
Cholesterol	60 mg	**Phosphorus**	290 mg
Sodium	580 mg		

Protein Hummus and Crisp Veggies

SERVES: 4 / **SERVING SIZE:** $^2/_3$ cup vegetables and $^2/_3$ cup hummus and egg mixture

4	hard boiled eggs
1⅓	cup prepared hummus
1	teaspoon dried dill
¾	ounce reduced-fat feta cheese, crumbled
1	medium green bell pepper, cut in strips
½	of a medium cucumber, sliced

1 Discard two of the egg yolks and finely chop remaining eggs. Spoon hummus into a shallow bowl, sprinkle with the dill, top with finely chopped eggs, and sprinkle with the feta. Serve with the bell pepper strips and cucumber slices.

EXCHANGES/CHOICES
½ starch, 1 vegetable, 1 lean meat, 1 fat

Calories	210	**Potassium**	280 mg
Calories from Fat	100	**Total Carbohydrate**	15 g
Total Fat	11 g	Dietary Fiber	6 g
Saturated Fat	2.5 g	Sugars	2 g
Trans Fat	0 g	**Protein**	13 g
Cholesterol	110 mg	**Phosphorus**	150 mg
Sodium	450 mg		

Creamy Chicken Corn Soup

SERVES: 4 / **SERVING SIZE:** 1 cup

1 Combine all ingredients except the cheese in a large saucepan. Bring just to a simmer over medium-high heat. Remove from heat.

2 Stir in the cheese until melted.

2 cups fat-free milk
2 cups cooked diced chicken
¾ cup frozen corn
1 (4.5-ounce) can chopped mild green chilies
½ teaspoon ground cumin
4 wedges light chipotle-flavored Swiss cheese spread (such as Laughing Cow)

EXCHANGES/CHOICES
½ starch, ½ skim milk, 3 lean meat

Calories	230	**Potassium**	480 mg
Calories from Fat	45	**Total Carbohydrate**	15 g
Total Fat	5 g	Dietary Fiber	1 g
Saturated Fat	2 g	Sugars	8 g
Trans Fat	0 g	**Protein**	29 g
Cholesterol	70 mg	**Phosphorus**	310 mg
Sodium	470 mg		

Chicken, Pasta, and Spinach Soup, PAGE 63

Chicken, Pasta, and Spinach Soup

SERVES: 4 / **SERVING SIZE:** 1¼ cups soup plus 2 teaspoons cheese

1 In a medium saucepan, combine the broth and tomatoes and their liquid and bring to a boil over high heat. Stir in the pasta, return to a boil, reduce heat, cover, and simmer 6 minutes or until pasta is just tender.

2 Remove from heat and stir in the remaining ingredients, except the cheese. Let stand, covered, 5 minutes to absorb flavors and heat through. Serve topped with cheese.

1 (14-ounce) can reduced-sodium chicken broth

1 (14.5-ounce) can no-salt-added diced tomatoes

2 ounces whole grain or multigrain pasta (such as rotini)

2 cups cooked diced chicken breast

1 cup packed baby spinach

¼ cup chopped fresh basil

1 tablespoon extra-virgin olive oil

¼ teaspoon salt

2 tablespoons grated Parmesan cheese

EXCHANGES/CHOICES
1 starch, 3 lean meat, 1 fat

Calories	260	**Potassium**	580 mg
Calories from Fat	90	**Total Carbohydrate**	15 g
Total Fat	10 g	Dietary Fiber	3 g
Saturated Fat	2.5 g	Sugars	4 g
Trans Fat	0 g	**Protein**	26 g
Cholesterol	60 mg	**Phosphorus**	250 mg
Sodium	430 mg		

Sausage, Bean, and Carrot Soup

SERVES: 4 / **SERVING SIZE:** 1¼ cups

1	teaspoon canola oil
8	ounces Italian turkey sausage, hot or mild, casings removed
1	cup chopped green onion
⅓	(15-ounce) can no-salt-added navy beans, rinsed and drained
1	cup sliced carrots
1½	cups water
1	(14.5-ounce) can no-salt-added diced tomatoes
½	teaspoon dried fennel or to taste
⅛	teaspoon dried pepper flakes
¼	cup chopped fresh parsley

1 Heat the oil in a large saucepan over medium-high heat. Add the sausage and cook 4 minutes or until browned, breaking up larger pieces while cooking. Add the remaining ingredients except the parsley. Bring to a boil over high heat. Reduce heat to medium low, cover, and simmer 15 minutes or until carrots are tender.

2 Remove from heat, stir in the parsley, and let stand, covered, 15–20 minutes to allow flavors to develop.

EXCHANGES/CHOICES
1 starch, 1 vegetable, 1½ lean meat

Calories	170	**Potassium**	640 mg
Calories from Fat	60	**Total Carbohydrate**	15 g
Total Fat	6 g	Dietary Fiber	5 g
Saturated Fat	2 g	Sugars	6 g
Trans Fat	0 g	**Protein**	13 g
Cholesterol	35 mg	**Phosphorus**	200 mg
Sodium	440 mg		

Tomato-Cilantro Soup

SERVES: 4 / **SERVING SIZE:** 1 cup soup plus ¼ cup avocado

1 Combine tomatoes and liquid, green chilies, carrots, water, and ⅛ teaspoon salt in a large saucepan. Bring to a boil over high heat, reduce heat to medium low, cover, and simmer 10 minutes. Remove from heat.

2 Using a potato masher, mash the tomato mixture to break up larger pieces. Stir in remaining ingredients, except the avocado. Top with equal amounts of the avocado. Serve immediately for peak flavors.

2 (14.5-ounce) cans no-salt-added stewed tomatoes, drained
1 (4-ounce) can chopped mild green chilies
1 (8-ounce) can sliced carrots, drained
½ cup water
⅛ teaspoon salt
½ cup chopped cilantro
1 tablespoon lime juice
1 tablespoon extra-virgin olive oil
2 teaspoons mild Louisiana hot pepper sauce (optional)
¼ teaspoon salt
1 ripe medium avocado, peeled and pitted

COOK'S TIP: If not serving immediately, you may cook it ahead, but do not stir in the "remaining ingredients" until time of serving.

EXCHANGES/CHOICES
3 vegetable, 2 fat

Calories	150	**Potassium**	750 mg
Calories from Fat	80	**Total Carbohydrate**	15 g
Total Fat	9 g	Dietary Fiber	6 g
Saturated Fat	1.5 g	Sugars	7 g
Trans Fat	0 g	**Protein**	2 g
Cholesterol	0 mg	**Phosphorus**	80 mg
Sodium	420 mg		

Black Bean–Green Pepper Soup

SERVES: 4 / **SERVING SIZE:** 1 cup

2 teaspoons canola oil, divided use

4 ounces smoked turkey sausage, diced

¾ cup diced green bell pepper or poblano chili pepper

2 cups water

1 (15-ounce) can no-salt-added black beans, rinsed and drained

½ cup diced tomato

⅛ teaspoon dried pepper flakes (optional)

¼ teaspoon salt

1 ounce shredded part-skim mozzarella cheese

1 Heat 1 teaspoon of the oil in a large saucepan over medium-high heat. Cook sausage 3 minutes or until beginning to brown, stirring frequently. Set aside on separate plate.

2 Heat the remaining 1 teaspoon oil. Cook the peppers 2–3 minutes or until beginning to brown on edges, stirring frequently. Add the water, beans, tomatoes, and pepper flakes. Bring to a boil over medium-high heat, reduce heat to medium low, cover, and cook 5–7 minutes or until peppers are tender. Remove from heat and add the sausage and salt. Cover and let stand 5 minutes to absorb flavors. Serve each topped with cheese.

EXCHANGES/CHOICES
1 starch, 2 lean meat

Calories	120	**Potassium**	420 mg
Calories from Fat	20	**Total Carbohydrate**	15 g
Total Fat	2.5 g	Dietary Fiber	4 g
Saturated Fat	1.0 g	Sugars	3 g
Trans Fat	0 g	**Protein**	10 g
Cholesterol	15 mg	**Phosphorus**	190 mg
Sodium	450 mg		

Asian Chicken, Cabbage, and Cilantro Salad

SERVES: 4 / **SERVING SIZE:** 2 cups

 In a small bowl, whisk together the dressing ingredients.

2 In a large bowl, combine all the salad ingredients. Pour the dressing over all and toss until well blended.

Dressing

2	tablespoons pourable sugar substitute
2	tablespoons white balsamic vinegar
2	tablespoons light soy sauce
1	tablespoon grated ginger
1	tablespoon canola oil

Salad

6	cups shredded green cabbage
1½	cups cooked chopped chicken or pork
3	ounces snow peas or sugar snaps, cut diagonally
½	medium cucumber, peeled and sliced
½	cup chopped green onions
2	ounces peanuts, toasted
½	cup chopped cilantro

EXCHANGES/CHOICES
3 vegetable, 3 lean meat, 2 fat

Calories	260	**Total Carbohydrate**	15 g
Calories from Fat	110	Dietary Fiber	5 g
Total Fat	13 g	Sugars	4 g
Saturated Fat	2.0 g	**Protein**	22 g
Trans Fat	0 g	**Phosphorus**	230 mg
Cholesterol	45 mg		
Sodium	370 mg		
Potassium	580 mg		

Layered Chicken Taco Salad

SERVES: 4 / **SERVING SIZE:** 3 cups

4 cups shredded romaine
½ cup diced tomatoes
1 (4-ounce) can chopped mild green chilies
2 cups chopped cooked chicken breast
1 teaspoon ground cumin
1 tablespoon lime juice (½ of a medium lime)
¼ cup chopped cilantro
2 ounces baked tortilla chips, coarsely crumbled
1 ounce reduced-fat sharp cheddar cheese, shredded
2 ounces sliced ripe olives (about 14 small pitted olives total)

1 Arrange lettuce on bottom of an 11 × 7-inch baking dish, top with the remaining ingredients in the order listed.

EXCHANGES/CHOICES
1 starch, ½ lean meat, ½ fat

Calories	120	**Potassium**	270 mg
Calories from Fat	45	**Total Carbohydrate**	15 g
Total Fat	5 g	Dietary Fiber	3 g
Saturated Fat	1.5 g	Sugars	1 g
Trans Fat	0 g	**Protein**	4 g
Cholesterol	<5 mg	**Phosphorus**	115 mg
Sodium	400 mg		

Chicken and Toasted Pecan Salad

SERVES: 4 / **SERVING SIZE:** 1 cup

1 Combine the mayonnaise, cumin, salt, and pepper flakes in a medium bowl. Stir in the chicken until well coated. Stir in the remaining ingredients.

¼ cup light mayonnaise
¼ teaspoon ground cumin
¼ teaspoon salt
⅛ teaspoon dried pepper flakes
2 cups cooked chopped chicken breast
1 oz chopped pecans, toasted
1 cup diced red bell pepper
½ cup finely chopped red onion
½ cup diced celery
⅓ cup dried cranberries

EXCHANGES/CHOICES
½ carbohydrate, 1 vegetable, 3 lean meat, 1 fat

Calories	250	**Potassium**	350 mg
Calories from Fat	100	**Total Carbohydrate**	15 g
Total Fat	11 g	Dietary Fiber	3 g
Saturated Fat	1.5 g	Sugars	10 g
Trans Fat	0 g	**Protein**	23 g
Cholesterol	60 mg	**Phosphorus**	200 mg
Sodium	280 mg		

Asian Chicken–Wild Rice Salad

1 cup water
1 cup quick-cooking wild rice
1 cup small broccoli florets
2 cups cooked diced chicken breast or turkey
½ cup diced red bell pepper
1½ tablespoons lite soy sauce
1 tablespoon pourable sugar substitute
1 tablespoon cider vinegar
1 tablespoon canola oil
2 teaspoons grated orange zest
¼ teaspoon dried pepper flakes
1 ounce chopped walnuts
½ cup chopped cilantro or mint

1 In a medium saucepan: bring water to boil over high heat, stir in the wild rice, reduce heat to medium low, cover, and simmer 3 minutes. Stir in the broccoli and cook 2 minutes longer or until broccoli is just tender-crisp. Drain in fine-mesh sieve and run under cold water to cool quickly. Shake off excess liquid.

2 Meanwhile, combine the remaining ingredients, except the cilantro, in a large bowl. Add the rice mixture and cilantro and stir until well blended.

EXCHANGES/CHOICES

1 starch, 1 vegetable, 3 lean meat

Calories	250	**Potassium**	360 mg
Calories from Fat	110	**Total Carbohydrate**	14 g
Total Fat	11 g	Dietary Fiber	2 g
Saturated Fat	1.5 g	Sugars	4 g
Trans Fat	0 g	**Protein**	25 g
Cholesterol	60 mg	**Phosphorus**	250 mg
Sodium	290 mg		

Turkey and Swiss Stuffed Eggs

SERVES: 4 / **SERVING SIZES:** 2 egg halves and 4 crackers

1 Remove the egg yolks from the eggs. Place egg yolks, mayonnaise, and mustard in a medium bowl. Using a fork, mash until well blended. Stir in the turkey, cheese, and basil. For a moister consistency, add 1–2 tablespoons fat-free milk to the mixture. Spoon equal amounts into the egg whites. Serve with crackers.

4 hard-boiled eggs, peeled and halved lengthwise

3 tablespoon light mayonnaise

2 teaspoons Dijon mustard

2 ounces low-sodium thinly sliced oven-roasted deli turkey slices, diced

2 thin-sliced reduced-fat Swiss cheese (1½ ounces total), finely chopped

1 tablespoon chopped fresh basil or parsley

16 reduced-fat triscuit-style crackers

EXCHANGES/CHOICES
1 starch, 2 medium-fat meat

Calories	210	**Potassium**	170 mg
Calories from Fat	90	**Total Carbohydrate**	15 g
Total Fat	10 g	Dietary Fiber	2 g
Saturated Fat	2.5 g	Sugars	2 g
Trans Fat	0 g	**Protein**	15 g
Cholesterol	200 mg	**Phosphorus**	235 mg
Sodium	470 mg		

Turkey, Greens, and Strawberry Almond Salad

SERVES: 4 / **SERVING SIZE:** 2½ cups

Salad

- 4 cups baby spinach leaves or torn Romaine leaves
- 4 cups torn fresh mustard greens or kale greens
- 4 ounces reduced-sodium cooked turkey breast, chopped
- 1 cup whole strawberries, quartered
- ½ cup (2 ounces) thinly sliced red onion
- 1½ ounces slivered almonds, toasted

Dressing

- 2 tablespoons canola oil
- 2 tablespoons white balsamic vinegar
- 1 tablespoon pourable sugar substitute
- ¼ teaspoon salt
- ¼ teaspoon dried red pepper flakes

 1 Combine the salad ingredients in a large bowl.

2 Whisk together the dressing ingredients in a small bowl, pour over the salad, and toss until well coated.

EXCHANGES/CHOICES

2 vegetable, ½ carbohydrate, 1 lean meat, 2 fat

Calories	210	**Potassium**	600 mg
Calories from Fat	120	**Total Carbohydrate**	14 g
Total Fat	13 g	Dietary Fiber	5 g
Saturated Fat	1 g	Sugars	8 g
Trans Fat	0 g	**Protein**	12 g
Cholesterol	10 mg	**Phosphorus**	160 mg
Sodium	360 mg		

Chunky Veggie Egg and Bean Salad

SERVES: 4 / **SERVING SIZE:** 1 cup

1 Combine the mayonnaise, vinegar, sugar substitute, and salt in a medium bowl. Add the remaining ingredients and stir until well blended.

- **3** tablespoons light mayonnaise
- **1** teaspoon cider vinegar
- **1** teaspoon pourable sugar substitute
- **½** teaspoon salt
- **1** (16-ounce) can no-salt added kidney beans, rinsed and drained
- **½** cup diced yellow or red bell pepper
- **½** cup diced celery
- **¼** cup finely chopped red onion
- **3** hard-boiled eggs, peeled and diced

EXCHANGES/CHOICES
1 starch, 1 vegetable, 1 medium-fat meat

Calories	190	**Potassium**	520 mg
Calories from Fat	70	**Total Carbohydrate**	15 g
Total Fat	8 g	Dietary Fiber	7 g
Saturated Fat	1.0 g	Sugars	2 g
Trans Fat	0 g	**Protein**	10 g
Cholesterol	160 mg	**Phosphorus**	210 mg
Sodium	460 mg		

Garbanzo-Feta Salad

SERVES: 4 / **SERVING SIZE:** 1 cup

1 (16-ounce) can no-salt-added garbanzo beans, rinsed and drained
¾ cup grape tomatoes, quartered
½ of a medium cucumber, diced
⅓ cup diced red onion
1 tablespoon cider vinegar
1 tablespoon extra-virgin olive oil
4 ounces reduced-fat feta

 Combine all ingredients, except feta, in a medium bowl. Gently stir in feta.

EXCHANGES/CHOICES
1 starch, 1 vegetable, 1 medium-fat meat

Calories	150	**Potassium**	290 mg
Calories from Fat	45	**Total Carbohydrate**	15 g
Total Fat	5 g	Dietary Fiber	4 g
Saturated Fat	0.5 g	Sugars	5 g
Trans Fat	0 g	**Protein**	8 g
Cholesterol	5 mg	**Phosphorus**	190 mg
Sodium	320 mg		

Grilled Sirloin and Blue Cheese Salad

SERVES: 4 / **SERVING SIZE:** 3½ cups salad, 3 tablespoons dressing, and 2½ ounces cooked beef

1. Sprinkle both sides of the beef with the black pepper and ⅛ teaspoon of the salt. Heat the oil in a large nonstick skillet or brush the grill pan with the oil. Cook the beef 4 minutes on each side or until slightly pink in center. Place on cutting board and let stand 10 minutes before thinly slicing against the grain.

2. Meanwhile, place the lettuce on a large serving platter or 4 individual dinner plates. Top with equal amounts of the bell pepper, onion, and sunflower seeds.

3. Whisk together the buttermilk, mayonnaise, garlic, and remaining ⅜ teaspoon salt. Spoon evenly over all. Arrange the tomatoes on top with the beef slices and sprinkle evenly with the blue cheese.

- 10 ounces lean boneless sirloin steak, about ¾-inch thick
- 1 teaspoon coarsely ground black pepper
- ½ teaspoon salt, divided use
- 1 teaspoon canola oil
- 8 cups torn romaine lettuce
- 1 cup diced green bell pepper
- ½ cup thinly sliced red onion (2 ounces total)
- 1 ounce hulled sunflower seeds, toasted
- ⅔ cup low-fat buttermilk
- 2 tablespoons light mayonnaise
- 1 medium garlic clove, minced (optional)
- ¾ cup grape tomatoes, halved
- 1 ounce reduced-fat blue cheese, crumbled

EXCHANGES/CHOICES
2 vegetable, 3 lean meat, 1½ fat

Calories	260	**Potassium**	810 mg
Calories from Fat	120	**Total Carbohydrate**	12 g
Total Fat	13 g	Dietary Fiber	4 g
Saturated Fat	2.5 g	Sugars	6 g
Trans Fat	0 g	**Protein**	24 g
Cholesterol	60 mg	**Phosphorus**	360 mg
Sodium	450 mg		

Ham and Edamame
Chop Salad, PAGE 77

Ham and Edamame Chop Salad

SERVES: 4 / **SERVING SIZE:** 2 cups

 1 In a small bowl, stir together the dressing ingredients.

2 In a large bowl, combine the salad ingredients, except the eggs. Cut the eggs in half, discard two yolk halves, and chop the remaining eggs. Add eggs to the salad with the dressing and toss until well coated.

Dressing

- ¼ cup light mayonnaise
- ¼ cup fat-free sour cream
- 1 medium garlic clove, minced
- 2 teaspoons cider vinegar
- 1 tablespoon dried dill weed

Salad

- 6 cups chopped Romaine lettuce
- 1 cup fresh shelled edamame
- 4 ounces extra-lean diced ham
- ½ medium cucumber, peeled and chopped
- ½ cup diced green bell pepper
- ⅓ cup diced red onion
- 2 ounces very thinly sliced reduced-fat Swiss cheese, torn in small pieces
- 2 large hard boiled eggs, peeled and halved

EXCHANGES/CHOICES

½ starch, 2 vegetable, 2 lean meat, ½ fat

Calories	200	**Potassium**	720 mg
Calories from Fat	80	**Total Carbohydrate**	15 g
Total Fat	9 g	Dietary Fiber	4 g
Saturated Fat	2 g	Sugars	5 g
Trans Fat	0 g	**Protein**	17 g
Cholesterol	70 mg	**Phosphorus**	310 mg
Sodium	530 mg		

Appetizers, Snacks & Beverages

DIPS AND SPREADS

Herbed Tomato-Olive Relish with Pita Chips
Cilantro-Lime Hummus with Tortilla Wedges
Jalapeño–Sour Cream Dip and Raw Veggies
Smoked Tuna Dip
Sweet-Hot Pepper Relish on Cream Cheese
Apples with Creamy Chocolate Peanut
    Butter Dip
Bulgur, Mint, and Tomatoes on
    Cucumber Rounds
Feta-Basil Crostini

CHIPS AND CRUNCHIES

Nutty, Seedy Cereal Snack Mix
Easy Poppin' Lemon-Dill Popcorn
Cinnamon-Apple Grahams
Ham and Avocado Cracker Stackers

BEVERAGES

Powerhouse Kiwi-Orange Juice
Steaming Cranberry-Raspberry Tea
Flurried Mocha

Herbed Tomato-Olive Relish with Pita Chips

SERVES: 4 / **SERVING SIZE:** ⅓ cup tomato mixture and 8 chips

2	whole-wheat pita rounds, halved crosswise and cut into 8 wedges each
14	pitted kalamata olives, chopped
1¼	cups sweet grape tomatoes, finely chopped (or 1 large tomato, seeded and finely chopped)
1	tablespoon chopped fresh basil or 1 teaspoon dried basil leaves
⅛	teaspoon dried pepper flakes (optional)
2	teaspoons extra-virgin olive oil
1	ounce reduced-fat feta, crumbled (¼ cup)

1 Preheat oven to 350°F.

2 Arrange the pita wedges on a large cookie sheet in a single layer. Bake 7 minutes or until just beginning to lightly brown. Cool completely.

3 Meanwhile, combine the remaining ingredients, except the feta, in a shallow bowl. Serve topped with feta. Serve with pita chips.

EXCHANGES/CHOICES
1 starch, 1 vegetable, 1 fat

Calories	140	**Potassium**	140 mg
Calories from Fat	70	**Total Carbohydrate**	15 g
Total Fat	7 g	Dietary Fiber	2 g
Saturated Fat	1.5 g	Sugars	1 g
Trans Fat	0 g	**Protein**	4 g
Cholesterol	5 mg	**Phosphorus**	80 mg
Sodium	420 mg		

COOK'S TIP: When tomatoes are not in season, sweet grape tomatoes are the most flavorful and pop with color . . . it's worth the chop!

Cilantro-Lime Hummus with Tortilla Wedges

SERVES: 12 / **SERVING SIZE:** 3 tablespoons hummus and 6 tortilla wedges

 1 Preheat the oven to 350°F.

2 Arrange the tortilla wedges on 2 large cookie sheets. Bake 8 minutes or until just beginning to lightly brown. Sprinkle evenly with ¼ teaspoon salt and cool completely.

3 Meanwhile, combine the avocado, beans, garlic, sour cream, cilantro, lemon juice, mustard, and cumin in a blender. Purée until smooth. Place in a medium bowl, stir in the tomatoes, oil, and ½ teaspoon salt. Serve with tortilla wedges.

Wedges
- **9** corn tortillas, cut into 8 wedges
- **¼** teaspoon salt

Hummus
- **2** ripe avocadoes, peeled and pit removed
- **½** (15-ounce) can no-salt-added navy beans, rinsed and drained
- **2** medium garlic cloves, peeled
- **½** cup fat-free sour cream
- **½** cup chopped cilantro
- **3** tablespoons lemon juice
- **2** teaspoons prepared mustard
- **½** teaspoon ground cumin
- **1** medium tomato, seeded and diced
- **1** tablespoon extra-virgin olive oil
- **½** teaspoon salt

EXCHANGES/CHOICES
1 starch, 1 fat

Calories	120	**Potassium**	240 mg
Calories from Fat	45	**Total Carbohydrate**	15 g
Total Fat	5 g	Dietary Fiber	4 g
Saturated Fat	1 g	Sugars	1 g
Trans Fat	0 g	**Protein**	3 g
Cholesterol	0 mg	**Phosphorus**	110 mg
Sodium	140 mg		

Jalapeño–Sour Cream Dip and Raw Veggies

½ cup low-fat buttermilk

⅓ cup light mayonnaise

⅓ cup fat-free sour cream

1 tablespoon water (optional)

2 medium jalapeños, seeded and finely chopped

1 medium garlic clove, minced

½ teaspoon ground cumin

¼ teaspoon salt

4 cups mixed raw vegetables (such as broccoli, cauliflower, red bell pepper strips, and sweet grape tomatoes)

 In a medium bowl, whisk together the salad dressing ingredients until smooth.

 Serve with raw vegetables.

EXCHANGES/CHOICES

2 vegetable, 1 fat

Calories	110	**Potassium**	440 mg
Calories from Fat	45	**Total Carbohydrate**	14 g
Total Fat	5 g	Dietary Fiber	3 g
Saturated Fat	1 g	Sugars	6 g
Trans Fat	0 g	**Protein**	4 g
Cholesterol	5 mg	**Phosphorus**	100 mg
Sodium	330 mg		

Smoked Tuna Dip

SERVES: 4 / **SERVING SIZE:** ¼ cup and 8 crackers

1 Place tuna in a fine mesh sieve, run under water, and drain. Using the back of a spoon or rubber spatula, press down to squeeze out excess liquid. Place in a small bowl with the remaining ingredients, except the crackers.

2 Serve immediately or cover and refrigerate up to 24 hours before serving. Serve with the crackers.

1 (5-ounce) can no-salt-added tuna packed in water
6 ounces fat-free cream cheese, softened
3 tablespoons light mayonnaise
1½–2 teaspoons liquid smoke
½ teaspoon Worcestershire sauce
¼ teaspoon garlic powder
32 reduced-sodium wheat crackers, such as Wheat Thins

COOK'S TIP: Great for lunch ... and enough protein, too! Serve with celery and cucumber slices alongside, if desired.

EXCHANGES/CHOICES
1 starch, 2 lean meat

Calories	170		**Potassium**	240 mg
Calories from Fat	50		**Total Carbohydrate**	15 g
Total Fat	6 g		Dietary Fiber	2 g
Saturated Fat	1 g		Sugars	3 g
Trans Fat	0 g		**Protein**	15 g
Cholesterol	20 mg		**Phosphorus**	320 mg
Sodium	510 mg			

Sweet-Hot Pepper Relish on Cream Cheese

SERVES: 4 / **SERVING SIZE:** 4 teaspoons relish mixture, 2 tablespoons cream cheese, and 3 crackers

2 tablespoons apricot fruit spread

1 medium jalapeño, finely chopped and seeded, if desired

⅓ cup finely chopped red bell pepper

⅛ teaspoon salt

1½ teaspoons pourable sugar substitute

1½ teaspoons balsamic vinegar

½ teaspoon grated orange zest (optional)

4 ounces fat-free cream cheese

12 cracked pepper water crackers

1 Combine the fruit spread, jalapeño, bell pepper, and salt in a small saucepan. Bring to a boil over medium heat, cook 1 minute. Remove from heat.

2 Stir in the sugar substitute, vinegar, and orange zest. Let stand to cool completely, about 15 minutes.

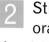

3 Serve over cream cheese. Serve with crackers.

EXCHANGES/CHOICES
1 starch, ½ lean meat

Calories	100	**Potassium**	130 mg
Calories from Fat	10	**Total Carbohydrate**	15 g
Total Fat	1.5 g	Dietary Fiber	1 g
Saturated Fat	0.5 g	Sugars	7 g
Trans Fat	0 g	**Protein**	6 g
Cholesterol	<5 mg	**Phosphorus**	190 mg
Sodium	340 mg		

Apples with Creamy Chocolate Peanut Butter Dip

SERVES: 4 / **SERVING SIZE:** ½ cup apple slices and 2 tablespoons peanut butter mixture

1 Combine the peanut butter and whipped topping in a medium microwave-safe bowl. Microwave on high 1 minute or until slightly melted. Whisk in remaining ingredients, except the apples.

2 Serve with apples.

3	tablespoons low-sodium less-sugar peanut butter
⅓	cup fat-free whipped topping
¼	cup water
1	tablespoon pourable sugar substitute
1	tablespoon cocoa powder
½	teaspoon vanilla extract
2	cups apple slices

EXCHANGES/CHOICES
1 fruit, 1 lean meat, 1 fat

Calories	120	**Potassium**	170 mg
Calories from Fat	60	**Total Carbohydrate**	15 g
Total Fat	7 g	Dietary Fiber	3 g
Saturated Fat	1.5 g	Sugars	10 g
Trans Fat	0 g	**Protein**	4 g
Cholesterol	<5 mg	**Phosphorus**	65 mg
Sodium	10 mg		

Bulgur, Mint, and Tomatoes on Cucumber Rounds, PAGE 87

Bulgur, Mint, and Tomatoes on Cucumber Rounds

SERVES: 4 / **SERVING SIZE:** ½ cup bulgur mixture and 8 cucumber slices

1. Bring water and bulgur to a boil in a medium saucepan over high heat. Reduce heat, cover, and simmer 12 minutes.

2. Meanwhile, combine the remaining ingredients, except the cucumber, in a medium bowl.

3. Drain bulgur in a fine-mesh sieve and run under cold water to cool quickly. Shake off excess liquid and stir into the tomato mixture.

4. Serve with cucumber slices.

⅓	cup dry, quick-cooking bulgur
1	cup water
1	cup finely chopped fresh mint
1	medium plum tomato, diced
1	tablespoon lemon juice
1½	tablespoons canola oil
1	tablespoon cider vinegar
¼	cup finely chopped red onion
⅛	teaspoon dried red pepper flakes
¼	teaspoon salt
32	cucumber slices (about ¼-inch thick each) (12 ounces total)

EXCHANGES/CHOICES
1 starch, 1 fat

Calories	110	**Potassium**	300 mg
Calories from Fat	45	**Total Carbohydrate**	15 g
Total Fat	5 g	Dietary Fiber	4 g
Saturated Fat	0.5 g	Sugars	3 g
Trans Fat	0 g	**Protein**	3 g
Cholesterol	0 mg	**Phosphorus**	70 mg
Sodium	110 mg		

Feta-Basil Crostini

SERVES: 4 / **SERVING SIZE:** 3 bread pieces, 1 tablespoon cream cheese mixture, 3 tablespoons feta, and ¼ cup tomatoes

4	ounces whole-grain or multigrain French bread, cut in 6 slices, then each cut in half crosswise
2	ounces fat-free cream cheese, softened
½	medium garlic clove, minced
2	tablespoons chopped fresh basil
3	ounces fat-free feta cheese
4	ounces tomatoes, diced

 Preheat oven to 350°F.

 Place bread slices on a baking sheet, bake 3 minutes on each side or until just lightly golden. Remove from oven and cool completely.

3 Meanwhile, mix cream cheese, garlic, and basil in a small bowl.

4 Spread the cream cheese mixture evenly over each bread slice, sprinkle evenly with the feta and top with the tomatoes.

EXCHANGES/CHOICES
1 starch, ½ lean meat

Calories	100	**Potassium**	170 mg
Calories from Fat	5	**Total Carbohydrate**	14 g
Total Fat	0.5 g	Dietary Fiber	2 g
Saturated Fat	0 g	Sugars	2 g
Trans Fat	0 g	**Protein**	8 g
Cholesterol	5 mg	**Phosphorus**	200 mg
Sodium	340 mg		

COOK'S TIP: There are 10 grams of protein in every serving! This may be served as a meatless entrée, if desired.

Nutty, Seedy Cereal Snack Mix

SERVES: 4 / **SERVING SIZE:** ½ cup

1 Heat a large skillet over medium-high heat. Add the almonds and pumpkin seeds and cook 3 minutes or until just beginning to lightly brown, stirring frequently. Place in a medium bowl.

2 Add the remaining ingredients to the almond mixture and toss until well blended.

1½	ounces sliced almonds
1½	ounces hulled pumpkin seeds
2	tablespoons dried cranberries
1	cup honey nut–flavored Chex-style cereal
⅛	teaspoon salt

EXCHANGES/CHOICES
1 starch, 2 fat

Calories	170	**Potassium**	180 mg
Calories from Fat	110	**Total Carbohydrate**	15 g
Total Fat	11 g	Dietary Fiber	3 g
Saturated Fat	1 g	Sugars	6 g
Trans Fat	0 g	**Protein**	6 g
Cholesterol	0 mg	**Phosphorus**	180 mg
Sodium	110 mg		

Easy Poppin' Lemon-Dill Popcorn

SERVES: 3 / **SERVING SIZE:** 2⅔ cups

1	tablespoon vegetable oil
⅓	cup yellow popcorn kernels
	Buttery pump spray
1	tablespoon grated lemon zest
1	teaspoon dried dill
¼	teaspoon salt

1 Combine the oil and popcorn kernels in a large saucepan, cover, and place over medium heat. When kernels begin popping, continue cooking 2 minutes or until the popping stops. Immediately remove cover and pump the butter spray 15 times over the popcorn, sprinkle with the remaining ingredients, and toss until well blended.

EXCHANGES/CHOICES
1 starch, 1½ fat

Calories	120	**Potassium**	70 mg
Calories from Fat	45	**Total Carbohydrate**	15 g
Total Fat	5 g	Dietary Fiber	3 g
Saturated Fat	1 g	Sugars	0 g
Trans Fat	0 g	**Protein**	2 g
Cholesterol	0 mg	**Phosphorus**	60 mg
Sodium	150 mg		

Cinnamon-Apple Grahams

SERVES: 4 / **SERVING SIZE:** 1 tablespoon peanut butter mixture, 2 graham crackers, and 2 tablespoons apple

1 Stir together the peanut butter, sugar substitute, and the cinnamon in a small bowl. Spread equal amounts on each cracker, top with the apple.

- **2** tablespoons plus 2 teaspoons low-sodium, 33% less sugar peanut butter
- **2** teaspoons pourable sugar substitute
- **⅛** teaspoon ground cinnamon
- **8** graham cracker squares (2½ inches each)
- **½** cup diced apple

EXCHANGES/CHOICES
1 starch, 1½ fat

Calories	130	**Potassium**	110 mg
Calories from Fat	60	**Total Carbohydrate**	15 g
Total Fat	7 g	Dietary Fiber	2 g
Saturated Fat	1.5 g	Sugars	7 g
Trans Fat	0 g	**Protein**	4 g
Cholesterol	0 mg	**Phosphorus**	60 mg
Sodium	70 mg		

Ham and Avocado Cracker Stackers

SERVES: 4 / **SERVING SIZE:** 4 stacks

2	teaspoons Dijon mustard
2	teaspoons light mayonnaise
16	reduced-fat Triscuit-style crackers
2	thin-sliced reduced-fat Swiss cheese
2	ounces shaved extra-lean ham, diced
½	ripe avocado, cut into 16 cubes
4	grape tomatoes, cut into four wedges

1 In a small bowl, combine the mustard and mayonnaise. Spoon equal amounts on each cracker (about ¼ teaspoon each). Top with cheese, ham, and avocado. Place the tomato alongside the avocado.

EXCHANGES/CHOICES
1 starch, 1 lean meat, ½ fat

Calories	140	**Potassium**	290 mg
Calories from Fat	45	**Total Carbohydrate**	15 g
Total Fat	5 g	Dietary Fiber	3 g
Saturated Fat	1 g	Sugars	1 g
Trans Fat	0 g	**Protein**	7 g
Cholesterol	10 mg	**Phosphorus**	160 mg
Sodium	390 mg		

Powerhouse Kiwi-Orange Juice

SERVES: 4 / **SERVING SIZE:** ¾ cup

 Combine all ingredients in a blender and purée until smooth.

3 ripe kiwi, peeled
1 cup orange juice
1 tablespoon lime juice
1 cup diet ginger ale

COOK'S TIP: One serving contains 2 grams of fiber and 130% daily requirement of Vitamin C!

EXCHANGES/CHOICES
1 fruit

Calories	70	**Potassium**	330 mg
Calories from Fat	0	**Total Carbohydrate**	15 g
Total Fat	0 g	Dietary Fiber	1 g
Saturated Fat	0 g	Sugars	12 g
Trans Fat	0 g	**Protein**	1 g
Cholesterol	0 mg	**Phosphorus**	30 mg
Sodium	20 mg		

Steaming Cranberry-Raspberry Tea

SERVES: 5 / **SERVING SIZE:** ¾ cup

2¼	cups cranberry raspberry juice
12	ounces diet ginger ale
¼	cup water
1	single tea bag
4	orange or lemon slices

1 Bring all ingredients, except the tea bag and fruit slices, to a boil over high heat in a medium saucepan. Remove from heat, add the tea bag, and "steep" for 3 minutes, dousing the tea bag up and down frequently. Remove tea bag. Serve with lemon or orange slices.

EXCHANGES/CHOICES
1 fruit

Calories	60	**Potassium**	110 mg
Calories from Fat	0	**Total Carbohydrate**	15 g
Total Fat	0 g	Dietary Fiber	0 g
Saturated Fat	0 g	Sugars	14 g
Trans Fat	0 g	**Protein**	0 g
Cholesterol	0 mg	**Phosphorus**	5 mg
Sodium	25 mg		

Flurried Mocha

SERVES: 6 / **SERVING SIZE:** ¾ cup

1 Combine all ingredients in a blender and purée until smooth. Serve immediately for peak volume and texture.

2 cups fat-free milk
⅔ cup fat-free half and half
¼ cup unsweetened cocoa powder
1½ tablespoons instant coffee granules
½ cup pourable sugar substitute
½ teaspoon vanilla extract
1 cup ice cubes

EXCHANGES/CHOICES
½ skim milk, ½ carbohydrate

Calories	80	**Potassium**	290 mg
Calories from Fat	10	**Total Carbohydrate**	15 g
Total Fat	1 g	Dietary Fiber	1 g
Saturated Fat	0.5 g	Sugars	11 g
Trans Fat	0 g	**Protein**	4 g
Cholesterol	<5 mg	**Phosphorus**	150 mg
Sodium	60 mg		

Side Salads and More

FRUIT

Pear-Cucumber Mint Salad

Mango Fruit Salad with Coconut

Fresh Nectarine-Kiwi Salad

Creamy Curry Pineapple Slaw

Apple-Cherry Pecan Chutney

GREENS

Sweet Pea and Bacon Salad

Chopped Salad with Creamy Mustard Dressing

Black Bean and Romaine Salad

Strawberry-Pear Salad with White
    Balsamic Dressing

Lime'd Edamame and Avocado Salad

Garbanzo, Green Bean, and Blue Cheese Salad

Lemon-Dill Potato, Tomato, and
    Cauliflower Salad

Tomato, Pasta, and Artichoke Salad

GRAINS

Rosemary Farro with Tomatoes
  and Feta Salad

Broccoli Raisin Couscous Salad

Fresh Corn Salad with Tomatoes and Basil

Mexican Rice Salad on Sliced Tomatoes

Pear-Cucumber Mint Salad

SERVES: 4 / **SERVING SIZE:** 1 cup

2	medium-firm pears, peeled, halved, cored, and thinly sliced
½	medium cucumber, peeled and thinly sliced
2	ounces thinly sliced red onion
¼–½	cup chopped fresh mint
2	teaspoons grated lemon rind
2	tablespoons lemon juice
1½	tablespoons pourable sugar substitute
⅛	teaspoon salt

 Combine all ingredients in a medium bowl and toss gently until well blended.

EXCHANGES/CHOICES

1 fruit

Calories	60	**Potassium**	200 mg
Calories from Fat	0	**Total Carbohydrate**	15 g
Total Fat	0 g	Dietary Fiber	3 g
Saturated Fat	0 g	Sugars	9 g
Trans Fat	0 g	**Protein**	1 g
Cholesterol	0 mg	**Phosphorus**	25 mg
Sodium	75 mg		

Mango Fruit Salad with Coconut

SERVES: 4 / **SERVING SIZE:** ½ cup

1 Combine all ingredients, except the coconut, in a medium bowl. Sprinkle with the coconut.

1 ripe medium mango, peeled, seeded, and chopped or 1 cup mango slices or cubes

⅓ cup fresh or frozen, thawed blueberries or raspberries

½ cup pineapple tidbits in own juice, drained

1 teaspoon grated lime or lemon rind (optional)

2 tablespoons lime or lemon juice

2 teaspoons pourable sugar substitute

¼ cup flaked sweetened coconut

EXCHANGES/CHOICES
1½ fruit, ½ fat

Calories	80	**Potassium**	140 mg
Calories from Fat	20	**Total Carbohydrate**	15 g
Total Fat	2 g	Dietary Fiber	2 g
Saturated Fat	1.5 g	Sugars	14 g
Trans Fat	0 g	**Protein**	1 g
Cholesterol	0 mg	**Phosphorus**	15 mg
Sodium	15 mg		

Fresh Nectarine-Kiwi Salad

SERVES: 4 / **SERVING SIZE:** ¾ cup

1 cup sliced nectarines, peaches, or mango
½ cup banana slices
2 ripe medium kiwi, peeled and cut in 8 wedges
1 medium jalapeño, seeded (if desired) and finely chopped (optional)
2 teaspoons grated gingerroot
2 tablespoons orange juice
2 tablespoons chopped cilantro or mint (optional)

1 Combine all ingredients in a medium bowl.

EXCHANGES/CHOICES
1 fruit

Calories	60	**Potassium**	300 mg
Calories from Fat	5	**Total Carbohydrate**	15 g
Total Fat	0.5 g	Dietary Fiber	2 g
Saturated Fat	0 g	Sugars	11 g
Trans Fat	0 g	**Protein**	1 g
Cholesterol	0 mg	**Phosphorus**	30 mg
Sodium	0 mg		

Creamy Curry Pineapple Slaw

SERVES: 4 / **SERVING SIZE:** 1 cup

1 Combine the pineapple, mayonnaise, sugar substitute, curry, mustard, and salt in a medium bowl. Stir in the coleslaw and carrots.

- **1** (8-ounce) can pineapple tidbits in own juice, drained
- **⅓** cup light mayonnaise
- **1** tablespoon pourable sugar substitute
- **1** teaspoon curry powder
- **1** teaspoon prepared mustard
- **⅛** teaspoon salt
- **3** cups shredded coleslaw
- **1** cup matchstick carrots

EXCHANGES/CHOICES

1 vegetable, 1 fruit, 1 fat

Calories	105	**Potassium**	270 mg
Calories from Fat	45	**Total Carbohydrate**	15 g
Total Fat	5 g	Dietary Fiber	2 g
Saturated Fat	0.5 g	Sugars	9 g
Trans Fat	0 g	**Protein**	1 g
Cholesterol	<5 mg	**Phosphorus**	35 mg
Sodium	240 mg		

Apple-Cherry Pecan Chutney

SERVES: 4 / **SERVING SIZE:** ⅓ cup

1	ounce chopped pecans
1	teaspoon canola oil
½	cup diced onion
1	cup diced Granny Smith apple
¼	cup dried cherries
2	teaspoons balsamic vinegar
1	tablespoon packed brown sugar blend
1	tablespoon diet margarine

 Heat a medium skillet over medium heat. Cook the pecans 2–3 minutes or until beginning to lightly brown, stirring frequently. Remove pecans and set aside on separate plate. Heat the oil and cook the onions 3 minutes or until translucent.

 Add the apple, cherries, and vinegar, reduce heat to medium low, cover, and cook 2 minutes or until apples are just tender-crisp.

3 Remove from heat and stir in the remaining ingredients. Serve warm or cold.

EXCHANGES/CHOICES
1½ fruit, 1½ fat

Calories	130	**Potassium**	150 mg
Calories from Fat	70	**Total Carbohydrate**	15 g
Total Fat	8 g	Dietary Fiber	2 g
Saturated Fat	1 g	Sugars	12 g
Trans Fat	0 g	**Protein**	1 g
Cholesterol	0 mg	**Phosphorus**	30 mg
Sodium	25 mg		

Sweet Pea and Bacon Salad

SERVES: 4 / **SERVING SIZE:** About 1¾ cup salad plus 3 tablespoons dressing

 1 In a small bowl, whisk together the dressing ingredients.

2 Place equal amounts of the romaine on each of four salad plates. Top with equal amounts of the dressing, top with the peas, onion, and bacon.

Dressing
½ cup low-fat buttermilk
¼ cup light mayonnaise
1 teaspoon sugar
½ teaspoon cider vinegar

Salad
6 cups packed torn romaine lettuce
1 cup frozen green peas, thawed
½ cup diced red onion
4 center-cut slices turkey bacon, cooked and crumbled

EXCHANGES/CHOICES
½ starch, 1 vegetable, 1 medium-fat meat

Calories	140	**Potassium**	350 mg
Calories from Fat	60	**Total Carbohydrate**	13 g
Total Fat	7 g	Dietary Fiber	3 g
Saturated Fat	1.5 g	Sugars	6 g
Trans Fat	0 g	**Protein**	7 g
Cholesterol	15 mg	**Phosphorus**	135 mg
Sodium	440 mg		

Chopped Salad with Creamy Mustard Dressing

SERVES: 4 / **SERVING SIZE:** 2¼ cups

6 cups chopped romaine
1 medium cucumber, chopped
½ cup fresh or frozen, thawed edamame
⅓ cup finely chopped red onion
½ cup light mayonnaise
2 tablespoons water
1 medium clove garlic, minced
1 teaspoon prepared mustard
¼ teaspoon salt

1 Combine the lettuce, cucumber, edamame, and onion in a large bowl.

2 Stir together the mayonnaise, water, garlic, mustard, and salt in a small bowl. Add to the lettuce mixture and toss until well coated.

EXCHANGES/CHOICES
2 vegetable, ½ fat

Calories	180	**Potassium**	390 mg
Calories from Fat	110	**Total Carbohydrate**	15 g
Total Fat	12 g	Dietary Fiber	5 g
Saturated Fat	1 g	Sugars	4 g
Trans Fat	0 g	**Protein**	6 g
Cholesterol	10 mg	**Phosphorus**	70 mg
Sodium	430 mg		

Black Bean and Romaine Salad

SERVES: 4 / **SERVING SIZE:** 1½ cups salad and 3 tablespoons dressing

 Whisk together the dressing ingredients in a small bowl and set aside.

2 Combine all salad ingredients, except the beans, in a large salad bowl. Spoon equal amounts on four salad plates. Spoon equal amounts of the dressing on top and sprinkle with the black beans.

Dressing

⅓ cup picante sauce

⅓ cup light mayonnaise

2 teaspoons cider vinegar

1 medium garlic clove, minced

1 teaspoon pourable sugar substitute

1 tablespoon water

Salad

4 cups chopped romaine

1 medium cucumber, halved lengthwise and sliced

1 medium poblano chili pepper, thinly sliced and cut into 2-inch pieces

¼ cup diced red onion

½ (15.5-ounce) can no-salt-added black beans, rinsed and drained

EXCHANGES/CHOICES

1 vegetable, 1 fat

Calories	130	**Potassium**	65 mg
Calories from Fat	60	**Total Carbohydrate**	15 g
Total Fat	7 g	Dietary Fiber	5 g
Saturated Fat	0 g	Sugars	4 g
Trans Fat	0 g	**Protein**	4 g
Cholesterol	5 mg	**Phosphorus**	10 mg
Sodium	330 mg		

Strawberry-Pear Salad with White Balsamic Dressing, PAGE 107

Strawberry-Pear Salad with White Balsamic Dressing

SERVES: 4 / **SERVING SIZE:** 1½ cups salad and 2 tablespoons dressing

1 Place equal amounts of the spring greens on each of four salad plates. Top with equal amounts of the pear, strawberries, and onion.

2 In a small bowl, whisk together the dressing ingredients and spoon equal amounts over all. Sprinkle evenly with the cheese.

4 cups packed spring greens or baby spinach (4 ounces total)
½ medium firm pear, thinly sliced
1½ cups whole strawberries, quartered
½ cup thinly sliced red onion

Dressing
⅓ cup white balsamic vinegar
2½ tablespoons canola oil
½ teaspoon pourable sugar substitute
¼ teaspoon salt
¼ teaspoon coarsely ground black pepper
⅛ teaspoon dried pepper flakes
1 ounce crumbled reduced-fat blue cheese

EXCHANGES/CHOICES
1 fruit, 1 vegetable, 2 fat

Calories	160	**Potassium**	210 mg
Calories from Fat	90	**Total Carbohydrate**	15 g
Total Fat	10 g	Dietary Fiber	3 g
Saturated Fat	1.5 g	Sugars	8 g
Trans Fat	0 g	**Protein**	3 g
Cholesterol	<5 mg	**Phosphorus**	50 mg
Sodium	290 mg		

Lime'd Edamame and Avocado Salad

SERVES: 4 / **SERVING SIZE:** 1 cup

5	ounces fresh or frozen shelled edamame
1½	cups sweet grape tomatoes, quartered
½	cup diced celery
⅓	cup diced red onion
1	medium jalapeño, finely chopped
¼	cup chopped fresh cilantro
3	tablespoons lime juice
½	teaspoon salt
1	ripe medium avocado, peeled and chopped

 Combine all ingredients, except the avocado, in a medium bowl. Gently fold in the avocado until well blended.

EXCHANGES/CHOICES
2 vegetable, 1½ fat

Calories	130	**Potassium**	570 mg
Calories from Fat	60	**Total Carbohydrate**	13 g
Total Fat	7 g	Dietary Fiber	6 g
Saturated Fat	1 g	Sugars	3 g
Trans Fat	0 g	**Protein**	5 g
Cholesterol	0 mg	**Phosphorus**	100 mg
Sodium	330 mg		

Garbanzo, Green Bean, and Blue Cheese Salad

SERVES: 4 / **SERVING SIZE:** 1 cup

1 Bring water to a boil in a large saucepan, add the beans, and cook 1½ minutes or until just tender-crisp. Drain in a colander and run under cold water to cool quickly and stop cooking process. Drain well, shaking off excess liquid.

2 Place beans in a large bowl with remaining ingredients, except the cheese, and toss until well blended. Add the cheese and stir gently.

- **6** cups water
- **8** ounces green beans, trimmed and cut into 2-inch pieces
- **½** (16-ounce) can garbanzo beans, rinsed and drained
- **1** medium red bell pepper, thinly sliced and cut into 2-inch pieces
- **½** cup finely chopped red onion
- **¼** cup white balsamic vinegar
- **1** tablespoon pourable sugar substitute
- **1** tablespoon canola oil
- **1** teaspoon dried tarragon leaves
- **½** teaspoon salt
- **¼** teaspoon dried pepper flakes
- **1** ounce crumbled reduced-fat blue cheese

COOK'S TIP: Serve within 30 minutes for more pronounced flavors. Cover and refrigerate overnight for more marinated, slightly blended flavors.

EXCHANGES/CHOICES

1 starch, 1 vegetable, ½ medium-fat meat, ½ fat

Calories	120	**Potassium**	330 mg
Calories from Fat	50	**Total Carbohydrate**	15 g
Total Fat	5 g	Dietary Fiber	5 g
Saturated Fat	1 g	Sugars	6 g
Trans Fat	0 g	**Protein**	5 g
Cholesterol	5 mg	**Phosphorus**	100 mg
Sodium	290 mg		

Lemon-Dill Potato, Tomato, and Cauliflower Salad

SERVES: 4 / **SERVING SIZE:** 1 cup

4	cups water
8	ounces red potatoes, scrubbed and chopped (½-inch cubes)
4	ounces small cauliflower florets
1	cup grape tomatoes, quartered
⅓	cup diced red onion
1½	tablespoons extra-virgin olive oil
2	teaspoons grated lemon rind
2	tablespoons lemon juice
1	medium garlic clove, minced
1	tablespoon dried dill
½	teaspoon dried rosemary
¼	teaspoon salt
1½	ounces reduced-fat feta, crumbled

1. Bring the water to a boil over high heat in a large saucepan. Add the potatoes, return to a boil, and cook 2 minutes. Add the cauliflower, reduce heat, cover, and simmer 3 minutes or until potatoes are just tender. Place in a colander and run under cold water to cool quickly. Shake off excess liquid.

2. Meanwhile, combine the remaining ingredients, except the feta, in a medium bowl. Add the potato mixture and toss gently, yet thoroughly, until well blended. Add the feta and stir gently.

EXCHANGES/CHOICES
1 starch, 1½ fat

Calories	140	**Potassium**	510 mg
Calories from Fat	60	**Total Carbohydrate**	15 g
Total Fat	7 g	Dietary Fiber	3 g
Saturated Fat	1.5 g	Sugars	4 g
Trans Fat	0 g	**Protein**	4 g
Cholesterol	<5 mg	**Phosphorus**	100 mg
Sodium	250 mg		

Tomato, Pasta, and Artichoke Salad

SERVES: 4 / **SERVING SIZE:** ⅔ cup

 1 Cook the pasta according to the package directions, omitting any salt or fat.

2 Meanwhile, combine the remaining ingredients in a medium bowl.

3 Drain the pasta and run under cold water to cool quickly. Shake off excess liquid. Add to the tomato mixture. Toss gently until well blended.

2	ounces uncooked whole-grain rotini pasta
1	cup sweet grape tomatoes, quartered
½	(13.75-ounce) can artichoke heart quarters, drained
2	tablespoons canola oil
1	tablespoon white balsamic vinegar
2	tablespoons chopped fresh basil
1	medium garlic clove, minced
¼	teaspoon salt

EXCHANGES/CHOICES
1 starch, 1 vegetable, 1 fat

Calories	140	**Potassium**	280 mg
Calories from Fat	70	**Total Carbohydrate**	14 g
Total Fat	8 g	Dietary Fiber	2 g
Saturated Fat	0.5 g	Sugars	2 g
Trans Fat	0 g	**Protein**	4 g
Cholesterol	0 mg	**Phosphorus**	80 mg
Sodium	240 mg		

Rosemary Farro with Tomatoes and Feta Salad

SERVES: 4 / **SERVING SIZE:** ⅔ cup

1½	cups water
2	ounces (⅓ cup) dry farro
1	cup diced tomato
½	cup diced cucumber
¼	cup finely chopped red onion
½	cup finely chopped fresh parsley or mint
1	teaspoon chopped fresh rosemary or ¼ teaspoon dried rosemary, crumbled
1	teaspoon grated lemon zest
2	tablespoons lemon juice
1	tablespoon canola oil
⅛	teaspoon salt
⅛	teaspoon dried pepper flakes
2	ounces reduced-fat feta

1 Bring the water to a boil in a small saucepan over high heat. Stir in the farro, return to a boil, reduce heat, cover, and simmer 15 minutes or until just tender. Drain in a fine-mesh sieve and run under cold water to cool quickly. Shake off excess liquid.

2 Meanwhile, combine the remaining ingredients, except the cheese, in a medium bowl. Stir in the farro and gently stir in the cheese.

EXCHANGES/CHOICES
1 starch, ½ meat, ½ fat

Calories	120	**Potassium**	180 mg
Calories from Fat	45	**Total Carbohydrate**	14 g
Total Fat	5 g	Dietary Fiber	2 g
Saturated Fat	1.5 g	Sugars	2 g
Trans Fat	0 g	**Protein**	6 g
Cholesterol	<5 mg	**Phosphorus**	20 mg
Sodium	260 mg		

Broccoli Raisin Couscous Salad

SERVES: 4 / **SERVING SIZE:** ½ cup

1 Bring the water to a boil in a small saucepan. Stir in the couscous. Remove from heat, cover, and let stand 5 minutes.

2 Meanwhile, combine the remaining ingredients in a medium bowl and set aside.

3 Fluff the couscous with a fork, place couscous on a sheet of foil or baking sheet in a thin layer, and let stand 5 minutes to cool quickly. Stir into the broccoli mixture. Let stand 30 minutes to develop flavors.

⅓ cup water
⅓ cup uncooked whole-wheat couscous
1 cup small broccoli florets (about ½-inch pieces)
½ cup diced red bell pepper
¼ cup finely chopped red onion
1 ounce pine nuts or slivered almonds, toasted
2 tablespoons raisins
1 tablespoon canola oil
2 teaspoons pourable sugar substitute
2 teaspoons cider vinegar
¼ teaspoon salt
⅛ teaspoon dried pepper flakes

COOK'S TIP: For an even quicker cooling process, place the hot couscous in a fine-mesh sieve and run under cold water. Shake off excess liquid. Be sure to use a fine-mesh sieve, otherwise the couscous will slip though the holes.

EXCHANGES/CHOICES
1 starch, 1 vegetable, 1 fat

Calories	130	**Potassium**	160 mg
Calories from Fat	55	**Total Carbohydrate**	15 g
Total Fat	6 g	Dietary Fiber	2 g
Saturated Fat	1 g	Sugars	3 g
Trans Fat	0 g	**Protein**	3 g
Cholesterol	0 mg	**Phosphorus**	40 mg
Sodium	90 mg		

Fresh Corn Salad with Tomatoes and Basil, PAGE 115

Fresh Corn Salad with Tomatoes and Basil

SERVES: 4 / **SERVING SIZE:** ¾ cup

1 Bring water to a boil in a large saucepan over high heat. Add the corn, reduce heat to medium, and cook, covered, 8 minutes, or until tender-crisp when pierced with a fork. Drain in colander and run under cold water to cool quickly.

2 Meanwhile, combine remaining ingredients in a medium bowl. Cut the corn off the cobb and add to the tomato mixture. Toss gently until well blended.

- 4 small ears of corn, silks and husks removed
- ¾ cup grape tomatoes, halved
- 2 tablespoons chopped fresh basil leaves
- ½ teaspoon salt
- 2 tablespoons extra-virgin olive oil
- 1 tablespoon cider vinegar

EXCHANGES/CHOICES
1 starch, 1½ fat

Calories	130	**Potassium**	280 mg
Calories from Fat	70	**Total Carbohydrate**	15 g
Total Fat	8 g	Dietary Fiber	2 g
Saturated Fat	1 g	Sugars	5 g
Trans Fat	0 g	**Protein**	3 g
Cholesterol	0 mg	**Phosphorus**	70 mg
Sodium	210 mg		

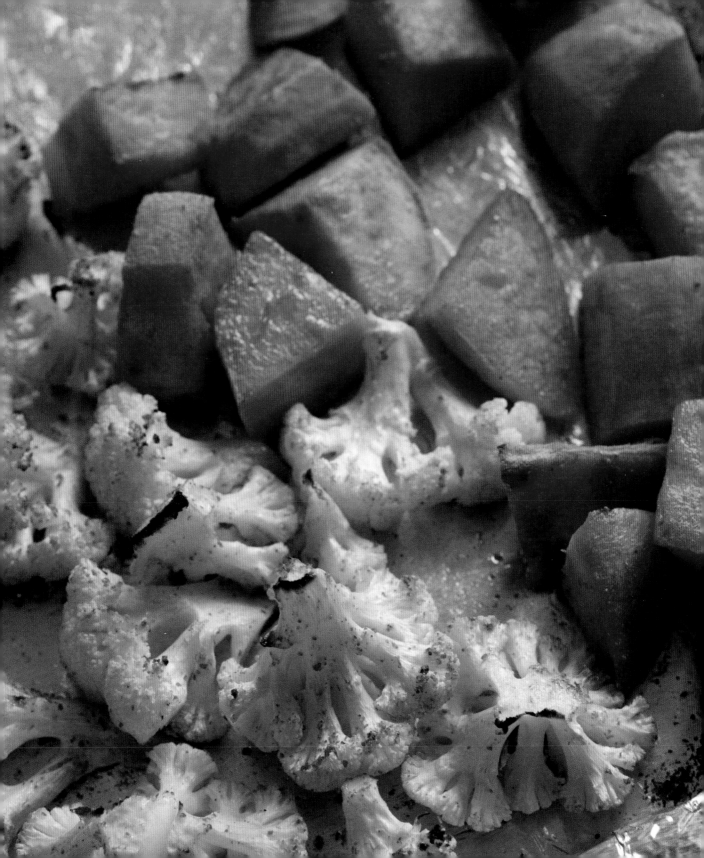

Mexican Rice Salad on Sliced Tomatoes

SERVES: 4 / **SERVING SIZE:** ½ cup rice mixture and 1 tomato slice

1. Combine all the ingredients, except the tomatoes, in a medium bowl.

2. Arrange a tomato slice on each of four salad plates. Spoon equal amounts of the rice mixture on top of each tomato slice.

- **1** cup cooked brown rice, chilled
- **½** cup diced cucumber
- **½** (4-ounce) can chopped mild green chilies
- **8** pitted ripe olives, chopped
- **¼** cup chopped cilantro
- **1** tablespoon cider vinegar
- **1** tablespoon extra-virgin olive oil
- **1** ounce shredded, reduced-fat sharp cheddar cheese
- **¼** teaspoon salt
- **6** ounces tomato, cut in 4 slices

COOK'S TIP: This is a great way to use leftover rice.

EXCHANGES/CHOICES
1 starch, 1 fat

Calories	130	**Potassium**	170 mg
Calories from Fat	50	**Total Carbohydrate**	15 g
Total Fat	6 g	Dietary Fiber	2 g
Saturated Fat	1.5 g	Sugars	2 g
Trans Fat	0 g	**Protein**	4 g
Cholesterol	<5 mg	**Phosphorus**	95 mg
Sodium	280 mg		

Entrées

POULTRY

Smothered Chicken and Potatoes

Cajun Chicken Stew

Cheddar-Sauced Chicken and Veggies

Smothered Picante Chicken with Black Beans

Saucy Chicken and Peppers

Chicken and Asparagus Wild Rice

Creamy Curried Chicken and Broccoli

Chicken, Zucchini, and Pasta with Feta

Chicken and Potato-Squash Skillet Casserole

Turkey Sausage and Vegetable Soup
    with Sage

Sausage and Cabbage Skillet

MEATLESS

Stuffed Portobellos with Spinach and Pine Nuts

Italian Veggie and Pasta Toss

Eggplant-Basil Rounds

Zucchini Ribbon Feta Pasta

SEAFOOD

Baked Fish with Lemon Panko Topping

Cornmeal-Crusted Fish Strips with Creamy
  Honey Mustard Sauce

Cod with Avocado Corn Salsa Salad

Grilled Tuna Steaks and Minted Cucumber
  Bulgur

Grilled Salmon, Grilled Veggie Quinoa

Spicy Shrimp and Tomato Pasta Toss

Scallops and Shallots on Snow Peas

BEEF

Beef Sirloin with Shallot-Mushroom Sauce

Beef Kabobs with Potatoes and Soy Balsamic
  Sauce

Sweet Home Beef and Veggie Pot Roast

Italian Veggie Smothered Beef Patties

Beef and Corn-Stuffed Skillet Peppers

Chili with Sausage and Beans

Blue Cheese Beef and Noodle Toss

PORK

Pork Tenderloin with Pineapple-Horseradish
  Sauce
Pork Tenderloin with Chipotle-Orange Veggies
Pork Chops with Broccoli Almond Rice
Grilled Pork and Sweet Potato Kabobs

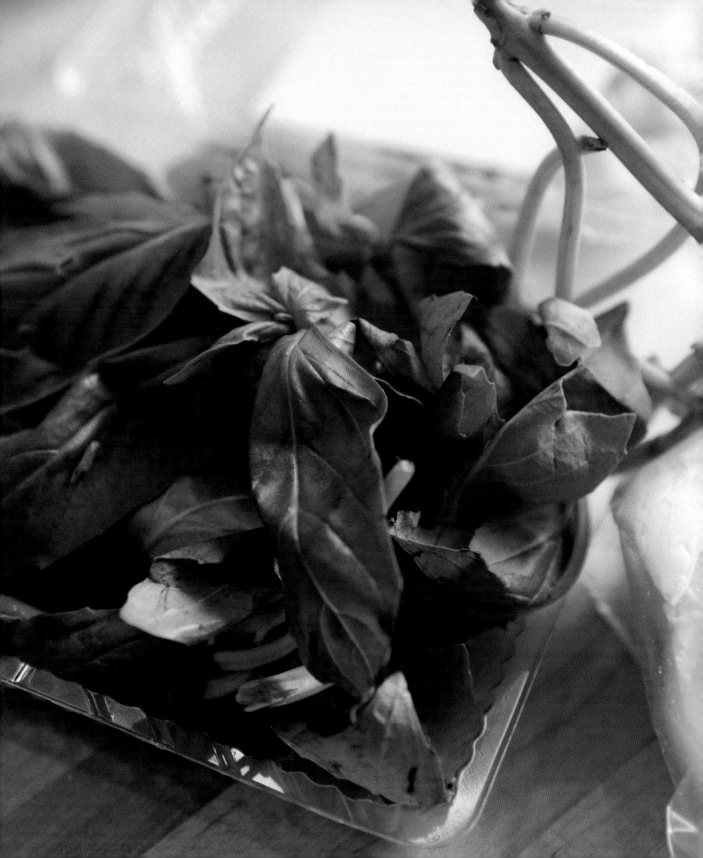

Smothered Chicken and Potatoes

SERVES: 4 / **SERVING SIZE:** 3 ounces cooked chicken and ¾ cup potato mixture

1   tablespoon flour
1   tablespoon canola oil
4   skinless, boneless chicken thighs, trimmed of fat (1 pound total)
1   cup reduced-sodium chicken broth
1   teaspoon dried thyme leaves
2   dried bay leaves
12 ounces small new potatoes, about 1-inch in diameter or larger new potatoes, cut in ½ inch wedges
¼   teaspoon plus ⅛ teaspoon salt

1 Heat a medium nonstick skillet over medium-high heat. Add the flour and cook 4 minutes or until beginning to turn golden, stirring constantly, and set aside on separate plate.

2 Heat the oil over medium-high heat. Add the chicken and cook 2 minutes on each side or until beginning to lightly brown.

3 Meanwhile, in a small bowl, whisk together the flour and ¼ cup of the broth until smooth. Whisk in the remaining broth with the thyme and pour over the chicken; add the bay leaves. Reduce heat to medium low, cover, and simmer 15 minutes. Add potatoes and ⅛ teaspoon salt, cover, and continue cooking 20–25 minutes or until potatoes are tender. Season with remaining ¼ teaspoon salt.

EXCHANGES/CHOICES
1 starch, 3 lean meat, ½ fat

Calories	240	**Potassium**	610 mg
Calories from Fat	70	**Total Carbohydrate**	15 g
Total Fat	8 g	Dietary Fiber	0 g
Saturated Fat	1.5 g	Sugars	1 g
Trans Fat	0 g	**Protein**	24 g
Cholesterol	135 mg	**Phosphorus**	250 mg
Sodium	400 mg		

Cajun Chicken Stew

SERVES: 4 / **SERVING SIZE:** 1¼ cups

1 Heat 1 teaspoon of the oil in a Dutch oven over medium-high heat. Brown sausage (about 2–3 minutes) and set aside on separate plate.

2 To the pan residue, heat 1 teaspoon oil, brown the chicken 4 minutes, stirring occasionally. Add the remaining ingredients, except the oil, sausage, and salt. Bring just to a boil, reduce heat to medium low, cover, and simmer 30 minutes or until chicken is no longer pink in center, stirring occasionally. Gently stir in the sausage, remaining oil, and salt, and remove from heat. Let stand, covered, 15 minutes to absorb flavors. Serve in shallow bowls.

2 tablespoons extra-virgin olive oil, divided use

4 ounces smoked turkey sausage, thinly sliced

1 medium green pepper, 1-inch chunks (4 ounces)

⅔ cup diced onion

2 medium garlic cloves, minced

1 pound boneless, skinless chicken thighs, trimmed of fat and cut into bite-size pieces

5 ounces fresh or frozen cut okra

2 dried bay leaves

1 teaspoon dried thyme leaves

1 (14.5-ounce) can no-salt-added stewed tomatoes

¼ teaspoon salt

EXCHANGES/CHOICES
3 vegetable, 4 lean meat, 1 fat

Calories	310	**Potassium**	780 mg
Calories from Fat	140	**Total Carbohydrate**	14 g
Total Fat	15 g	Dietary Fiber	3 g
Saturated Fat	2.5 g	Sugars	6 g
Trans Fat	0 g	**Protein**	31 g
Cholesterol	130 mg	**Phosphorus**	330 mg
Sodium	430 mg		

Cheddar-Sauced Chicken and Veggies

SERVES: 4 / **SERVING SIZE:** 3 ounces cooked chicken, ¾ cup vegetables, and ¼ cup sauce

2   cups fresh cauliflower florets, about ¾-inch pieces

1   cup sliced carrots

4   ounces red potatoes cut into ½-inch cubes

2   tablespoons canola oil, divided use

8   chicken tenderloins, about 1¼ pounds total, rinsed and patted dry

¼   teaspoon smoked paprika

¼   teaspoon black pepper

½   teaspoon salt, divided use

1   tablespoon flour

1   cup fat-free milk

1½   ounces reduced-fat sharp cheddar cheese, shredded

⅛   teaspoon cayenne pepper (optional)

     Pinch (or dash) ground nutmeg

1. Preheat oven 425°F.

2. Line a baking sheet with foil. Place the cauliflower, carrots, and potatoes on the foil, drizzle with 1 tablespoon of the oil, and toss until well coated. Arrange in a single layer. Place the chicken around the vegetables and sprinkle paprika and black pepper evenly over all. Bake 15–18 minutes or until chicken is no longer pink in center, stirring vegetables after 10 minutes.

3. Remove from oven, sprinkle with ¼ teaspoon salt, fold up corners of the foil, and seal, allowing it to steep for 5 minutes.

4. Meanwhile, heat the remaining 1 tablespoon oil in a medium saucepan over medium-low heat. Whisk in the flour until smooth. Gradually whisk in the milk until smooth. Cook over medium heat until thickened, stirring frequently. Remove from heat, stir in the cheese, the remaining ¼ teaspoon salt, and cayenne.

5. Place chicken in center of platter. Arrange veggies around chicken with any accumulated juices. Spoon sauce over the chicken and sprinkle lightly with nutmeg.

EXCHANGES/CHOICES

½ starch, 1 vegetable, 5 lean meat, 1 fat

Calories	330	**Potassium**	1000 mg
Calories from Fat	120	**Total Carbohydrate**	15 g
Total Fat	13 g	Dietary Fiber	3 g
Saturated Fat	2.5 g	Sugars	6 g
Trans Fat	0 g	**Protein**	37 g
Cholesterol	100 mg	**Phosphorus**	480 mg
Sodium	510 mg		

COOK'S TIP: May add 2 tablespoons additional milk to the sauce at the end, for a thinner sauce consistency.

Smothered Picante Chicken with Black Beans

SERVES: 4 / **SERVING SIZE:** 3 ounces cooked chicken and ½ cup bean mixture

1 Heat 1 teaspoon of the oil in a large non-stick skillet over medium-high heat. Sprinkle both sides of the chicken with cumin and cook 2 minutes, turn, and place the poblano peppers and black beans around the chicken pieces. Spoon equal amounts of the picante sauce and green chilies on top of each chicken breast.

2 Cover and reduce heat to medium low and cook 12–15 minutes or until chicken is no longer pink in center. Serve in shallow bowls, drizzle evenly with remaining 2 teaspoons oil, top with cheese, and serve with lime wedges.

- **1** tablespoon extra-virgin olive oil, divided use
- **4** boneless, skinless chicken breasts, rinsed and patted dry (1 pound total), flattened to ½-inch thickness
- **1** teaspoon ground cumin
- **2** medium poblano chilies, diced
- **10** ounces no-salt-added black beans, rinsed and drained
- **½** cup picante sauce
- **1** (4-ounce) can chopped mild green chilies
- **2** ounces shredded part-skim mozzarella (½ cup)
- **1** medium lime, quartered

EXCHANGES/CHOICES
1 starch, 4 lean meat, ½ fat

Calories	280	**Potassium**	740 mg
Calories from Fat	70	**Total Carbohydrate**	15 g
Total Fat	8 g	Dietary Fiber	6 g
Saturated Fat	2.5 g	Sugars	2 g
Trans Fat	0 g	**Protein**	34 g
Cholesterol	75 mg	**Phosphorus**	360 mg
Sodium	520 mg		

Saucy Chicken and Peppers

SERVES: 4 / **SERVING SIZE:** 1 drumstick, 1 thigh, and ⅔ cup pepper mixture

1	teaspoon canola oil
4	chicken thighs with bone in, skin removed, and trimmed of fat
4	chicken drumsticks, skin removed
2	medium green bell peppers, cut into thin strips
4	ounces sliced mushrooms
1	medium onion, cut in 8 wedges
1	cup water
¼	cup tomato paste
2½	tablespoons balsamic vinegar
1	teaspoon garlic powder
1	teaspoon Worcestershire sauce
½	teaspoon salt

1 Heat the oil in a large nonstick skillet over medium-high heat. Brown the chicken pieces 8 minutes, turning frequently. Add the peppers, mushrooms, and onions.

2 In a small bowl, whisk together the remaining ingredients, except the salt. Pour over all. Bring to a boil over medium-high heat, reduce heat, cover, and simmer 55 minutes or until no longer pink in center, turning occasionally. Remove the chicken pieces from the skillet and place in a large shallow pasta bowl.

3 Add the salt to the pepper mixture, bring to a boil over medium-high heat, and boil 6 minutes or until slightly thickened. Pour over chicken. Serve in shallow bowls.

EXCHANGES/CHOICES
3 vegetable, 4½ lean meat

Calories	280	**Potassium**	940 mg
Calories from Fat	70	**Total Carbohydrate**	15 g
Total Fat	8 g	Dietary Fiber	3 g
Saturated Fat	2 g	Sugars	10 g
Trans Fat	0 g	**Protein**	36 g
Cholesterol	160 mg	**Phosphorus**	410 mg
Sodium	510 mg		

Chicken and Asparagus Wild Rice

SERVES: 4 / **SERVING SIZE:** 1¼ cups

1 In a large nonstick skillet, bring water to a boil over medium-high heat, add the rice, reduce to medium-low heat, cover, and cook 5 minutes. Drain in fine-mesh sieve and set aside in separate bowl.

2 Heat 1 tablespoon of the oil in the skillet over medium heat. Add the mushrooms and cook 4 minutes or until just beginning to lightly brown, stirring occasionally. Stir in the garlic and cook 15 seconds, stirring constantly. Stir in the asparagus to the mushrooms, cover, and cook 3 minutes or until asparagus is tender-crisp. Stir in chicken, tomatoes, rice, and basil and cook 2 minutes or until heated. Stir in salt and remaining 1 tablespoon oil.

- **1** cup water
- **1** cup quick-cooking wild rice
- **2** tablespoons extra-virgin olive oil, divided use
- **4** ounces whole mushrooms, wiped clean with a damp cloth and quartered
- **1** medium garlic clove, minced
- **4** ounces asparagus spears, trimmed and cut into 2-inch pieces
- **2** cups cooked chopped chicken breasts
- **¾** cup sweet grape tomatoes, quartered
- **¼–⅓** cup chopped fresh basil
- **½** teaspoon salt

EXCHANGES/CHOICES
½ starch, 2 vegetable, 3½ lean meat

Calories	250	**Potassium**	450 mg
Calories from Fat	90	**Total Carbohydrate**	15 g
Total Fat	10 g	Dietary Fiber	2 g
Saturated Fat	1.5 g	Sugars	2 g
Trans Fat	0 g	**Protein**	25 g
Cholesterol	60 mg	**Phosphorus**	250 mg
Sodium	260 mg		

Creamy Curried Chicken and Broccoli

SERVES: 4 / **SERVING SIZE:** 1 cup

1 cup water
3 cups small broccoli florets
2 cups cooked chopped chicken breasts
½ (10.75-ounce) can 98% fat-free cream of chicken soup
¾ cup nonfat Greek yogurt
¼ cup light mayonnaise
¼ cup water
1 teaspoon curry powder
1 ounce shredded reduced-fat sharp cheddar cheese
¼ cup panko breadcrumbs, lightly toasted

1 Preheat to 350°F.

2 In a medium nonstick skillet, bring the water and broccoli to a boil over medium-high heat. Reduce heat, cover, and simmer 3–4 minutes or until tender. Drain well, shaking off excess liquid. Return broccoli to skillet or place in bottom of an 11 × 7-inch baking pan. Sprinkle chicken evenly over all.

3 In a medium bowl, stir together the soup, yogurt, mayonnaise, water, and curry. Spoon evenly over the chicken. Sprinkle with the cheese and top with the breadcrumbs.

4 Bake 22 minutes or until cheese is melted.

EXCHANGES/CHOICES
2 vegetable, 3 lean meat, ½ skim milk, 1 fat

Calories	280	**Potassium**	630 mg
Calories from Fat	100	**Total Carbohydrate**	14 g
Total Fat	11 g	Dietary Fiber	3 g
Saturated Fat	3 g	Sugars	5 g
Trans Fat	0 g	**Protein**	29 g
Cholesterol	70 mg	**Phosphorus**	300 mg
Sodium	420 mg		

COOK'S TIP: You don't have to pitch the remaining portion of the soup . . . simply place it in an airtight container and freeze it for a later use!

Chicken, Zucchini, and Pasta with Feta

SERVES: 4 / **SERVING SIZE:** 1½ cups

1 Cook the pasta according to package directions, omitting any salt or fat.

2 Meanwhile, heat 1 teaspoon of the oil in a medium nonstick skillet over medium-high heat. Cook the chicken 3 minutes, stirring frequently. (The chicken will be pink in center at this point.) Set aside on separate plate.

3 To skillet, add the zucchini, onion, and pepper flakes. Cook 6 minutes or until onions are lightly browned. Add the garlic and the chicken, cook 1–2 minutes or until chicken is no longer pink in center, stirring frequently. Remove from heat.

4 Stir in the drained pasta and remaining ingredients, except the feta. Top with the feta.

2	ounces uncooked whole-grain rotini pasta
2	tablespoons extra-virgin olive oil, divided use
12	ounces boneless, skinless chicken breasts, cut into bite-size pieces
1	medium zucchini, halved lengthwise and sliced
½	cup diced onion
⅛–¼	teaspoon dried pepper flakes
2	medium garlic cloves, minced
1	cup sweet grape tomatoes, quartered
¼	cup chopped fresh basil or 1 tablespoon and 1 teaspoon dried basil leaves
¼	teaspoon salt
1½	ounces reduced-fat feta, crumbled (½ cup)

EXCHANGES/CHOICES
1 starch, 3 lean meat, 1 fat

Calories	260	**Potassium**	610 mg
Calories from Fat	100	**Total Carbohydrate**	15 g
Total Fat	11 g	Dietary Fiber	3 g
Saturated Fat	2.5 g	Sugars	4 g
Trans Fat	0 g	**Protein**	23 g
Cholesterol	60 mg	**Phosphorus**	290 mg
Sodium	330 mg		

Chicken and Potato-Squash Skillet Casserole

SERVES: 4 / **SERVING SIZE:** 1 cup

1	tablespoon extra-virgin olive oil
1	pound boneless chicken breast, cut into 1-inch pieces
½	cup diced onion
1	cup diced red bell pepper
8	ounces red potato, thinly sliced
6	ounces yellow squash, trimmed and sliced
½	teaspoon dried thyme leaves
2	tablespoons water
2	tablespoons chopped parsley
½	teaspoon salt
¼	teaspoon black pepper
1½	ounces shredded reduced-fat sharp cheddar cheese

1. Heat 1 teaspoon of the oil in a medium nonstick skillet over medium-high heat. Cook the chicken 2–3 minutes or until barely pink inside. Set aside on separate plate.

2. Heat 1 teaspoon of the oil, cook the onions and pepper 2 minutes, stir in the potatoes, squash, thyme, water, chicken, and any accumulated juices. Bring to a boil over medium-high heat. Reduce heat to medium low, cover, and cook 10–12 minutes or until potatoes are tender. Remove from heat.

3. Stir in the parsley, salt, black pepper, and remaining 1 teaspoon oil. Sprinkle evenly with the cheese. Let stand 5 minutes, uncovered, to absorb flavors.

EXCHANGES/CHOICES
1 starch, 4 lean meat

Calories	260	**Potassium**	920 mg
Calories from Fat	80	**Total Carbohydrate**	15 g
Total Fat	9 g	Dietary Fiber	3 g
Saturated Fat	2.5 g	Sugars	4 g
Trans Fat	0 g	**Protein**	29 g
Cholesterol	80 mg	**Phosphorus**	370 mg
Sodium	420 mg		

Turkey Sausage and Vegetable Soup with Sage

SERVES: 4 / **SERVING SIZE:** 1¼ cups

1 Heat the oil in a large saucepan over medium-high heat. Brown the sausage, breaking up larger pieces while cooking. Add the onions, carrots, and celery. Cook 2 minutes, stirring frequently. Add the garlic and cook 15 seconds, stirring constantly. Add the mushrooms, broth, water, and sage. Bring to a boil over high heat. Reduce heat, cover, and simmer 15 minutes or until onions are tender.

2 Stir in the remaining ingredients.

1	teaspoon canola oil
6	ounces turkey breakfast sausage, removed from casing
¾	cup diced onion
1	cup matchstick carrots
½	cup thinly sliced celery
2	medium garlic cloves, minced
8	ounces sliced mushrooms
1	(14.5-ounce) can reduced-sodium chicken broth
½	cup water
2	tablespoons finely chopped fresh sage or 2 teaspoons dried rubbed sage
½	(15-ounce) can no-salt-added navy beans, rinsed and drained
¼	cup finely chopped fresh parsley
¼	teaspoon black pepper

COOK'S TIP: The aromas take over the kitchen!!

EXCHANGES/CHOICES
1 starch, 1 vegetable, 2 lean meat

Calories	200	**Potassium**	590 mg
Calories from Fat	90	**Total Carbohydrate**	15 g
Total Fat	10 g	Dietary Fiber	4 g
Saturated Fat	2 g	Sugars	3 g
Trans Fat	0 g	**Protein**	13 g
Cholesterol	70 mg	**Phosphorus**	200 mg
Sodium	330 mg		

Sausage and Cabbage Skillet

SERVES: 4 / **SERVING SIZE:** 1¾ cups

8	ounces mild or hot Italian turkey sausage, removed from casings
6	cups coarsely chopped green cabbage
1	cup diced green bell pepper
½	cup diced onion
½	cup sliced carrots
14.5	ounce can no-salt diced tomatoes
1	teaspoon dried caraway seeds
1	teaspoon sugar

1. Heat a Dutch oven coated with cooking spray over medium-high heat. Brown the sausage, about 3 minutes, stirring frequently, breaking up larger pieces. Stir in the cabbage, bell pepper, onions, and carrots and cook 5 minutes or until cabbage has wilted slightly, stirring frequently. Stir in the remaining ingredients, cover, reduce heat to medium low, and cook 10 minutes or until vegetables are tender.

EXCHANGES/CHOICES
3 vegetable, 1 lean meat, 1 fat

Calories	160	**Potassium**	670 mg
Calories from Fat	60	**Total Carbohydrate**	15 g
Total Fat	6 g	Dietary Fiber	4 g
Saturated Fat	2 g	Sugars	6 g
Trans Fat	0 g	**Protein**	12 g
Cholesterol	35 mg	**Phosphorus**	180 mg
Sodium	430 mg		

Stuffed Portobellos with Spinach and Pine Nuts

SERVES: 4 / **SERVING SIZE:** 1 stuffed cap

1. Preheat broiler.

2. Coat both sides of the mushroom caps with cooking spray and place on a foil-lined baking sheet. Broil 4 minutes on each side or until tender. Remove from heat, turn caps smooth side down, and set aside.

3. Meanwhile, heat a large nonstick skillet over medium-high heat. Add the pine nuts and breadcrumbs and cook 1–2 minutes or until just beginning to lightly brown, stirring frequently. Set aside on a separate plate. Stir in the basil and pepper flakes.

4. To skillet: heat 1 teaspoon of the oil over medium-high heat, tilting skillet to coat bottom lightly. Add the spinach and cook 1 minute or until slightly wilted, stirring constantly, using two utensils as you would a stir-fry. Remove from heat.

5. To assemble: spoon equal amounts (2 tablespoons) of the spaghetti sauce on each of the mushroom caps. Spoon equal amounts of the spinach on each. Top with the feta and equal amounts of pine nut mixture. Broil 1 minute or until lightly browned.

4	medium portobello mushroom caps, wiped clean with paper towels
2	ounces pine nuts
¼	cup panko breadcrumbs
2	teaspoons dried basil leaves
¼	teaspoon dried pepper flakes
1	teaspoon canola oil
6	cups packed fresh spinach, chopped (about 6 ounces)
½	cup spaghetti sauce
2½	ounces reduced-fat feta

EXCHANGES/CHOICES
3 vegetable, 1 medium-fat meat, 2 fat

Calories	200	**Potassium**	780 mg
Calories from Fat	120	**Total Carbohydrate**	15 g
Total Fat	14 g	Dietary Fiber	4 g
Saturated Fat	2.5 g	Sugars	5 g
Trans Fat	0 g	**Protein**	10 g
Cholesterol	10 mg	**Phosphorus**	200 mg
Sodium	460 mg		

Italian Veggie and Pasta Toss

SERVES: 4 / **SERVING SIZE:** 1 cup

2 ounces whole-grain rotini

2 teaspoons canola oil

6 ounces whole mushrooms, quartered

½ teaspoon dried oregano

4 ounces zucchini, quartered lengthwise and cut into 1-inch pieces

1 cup grape tomatoes, halved

1 medium garlic clove, minced

2 tablespoons capers

¼ teaspoon salt

2 ounces grated part-skim mozzarella cheese

4 teaspoons grated Parmesan

1 Cook pasta according to package directions.

2 Meanwhile, heat the oil in a large nonstick skillet over medium-high heat. Cook the mushrooms and oregano for 2 minutes or until just beginning to release juices, stirring constantly. Add the zucchini and cook 2 minutes. Stir in the tomatoes and garlic and cook 1 minute to heat through. Remove from heat, stir in the drained pasta, capers, and salt. Sprinkle with mozzarella and Parmesan.

EXCHANGES/CHOICES
1 starch, 1 medium-fat meat

Calories	140	**Potassium**	370 mg
Calories from Fat	50	**Total Carbohydrate**	15 g
Total Fat	6 g	Dietary Fiber	3 g
Saturated Fat	2 g	Sugars	4 g
Trans Fat	0 g	**Protein**	8 g
Cholesterol	10 mg	**Phosphorus**	175 mg
Sodium	340 mg		

Eggplant-Basil Rounds

SERVES: 4 / **SERVING SIZE:** 2 rounds

1 Preheat broiler.

2 Coat eggplant slices with cooking spray, arrange in a single layer on a baking sheet and broil 4 minutes on each side or until beginning to lightly brown.

3 Preheat oven to 350°F. Place eggplant in an 11 × 7-inch baking pan, spoon the spaghetti sauce over all. Top with the meat substitute, basil, pepper flakes, and sprinkle the mozzarella evenly over all. Bake 15–18 minutes or until bubbly. Remove from oven and sprinkle with the Parmesan cheese.

12	ounces eggplant, peeled, if desired, cut into 8 rounds
¾	cup spaghetti sauce
2	meat substitute patties, finely chopped, or 1 cup veggie crumbles, such as MorningStar Grillers
¼	cup chopped fresh basil
¼	teaspoon dried pepper flakes (optional)
1½	ounces shredded part-skim mozzarella cheese
2	tablespoons grated Parmesan cheese

EXCHANGES/CHOICES
2 vegetable, 2 lean meat

Calories	150	**Potassium**	580 mg
Calories from Fat	45	**Total Carbohydrate**	13 g
Total Fat	5 g	Dietary Fiber	6 g
Saturated Fat	2 g	Sugars	6 g
Trans Fat	0 g	**Protein**	14 g
Cholesterol	10 mg	**Phosphorus**	220 mg
Sodium	330 mg		

Zucchini Ribbon
Feta Pasta, PAGE 137

Zucchini Ribbon Feta Pasta

SERVES: 4 / **SERVING SIZE:** 1 cup

1 Using a vegetable peeler, cut the zucchini lengthwise into thin ribbons. Set aside.

2 Cook pasta according to package directions, omitting any salt or fat. Add the zucchini the last 15 seconds of cooking.

3 Meanwhile, combine the remaining ingredients, except the cheese, in a large bowl.

4 Drain the pasta, reserving 2 tablespoons of the pasta water. Shake off excess liquid. Add the pasta mixture and reserved 2 tablespoons water to the tomato mixture and toss until well blended. Add the cheese and toss gently.

1	medium zucchini
2	ounces whole-grain spaghetti noodles, broken in half
1	cup grape tomatoes, halved
¼	cup finely chopped green onion
2	ounces slivered almonds
2	tablespoons chopped fresh dill
1	tablespoon grated lemon zest
1	tablespoon canola oil
½	medium garlic clove, minced
¼	teaspoon salt
⅛ to ¼	teaspoon dried pepper flakes (optional)
2½	ounces reduced-fat feta or reduced-fat blue cheese

EXCHANGES/CHOICES
1 starch, 1 medium-fat meat, 1 fat

Calories	210	**Potassium**	380 mg
Calories from Fat	120	**Total Carbohydrate**	15 g
Total Fat	13 g	Dietary Fiber	4 g
Saturated Fat	2.5 g	Sugars	2 g
Trans Fat	0 g	**Protein**	10 g
Cholesterol	10 mg	**Phosphorus**	200 mg
Sodium	380 mg		

Baked Fish with Lemon Panko Topping

SERVES: 4 / **SERVING SIZE:** 3 ounces cooked fish and about ½ cup topping

4 (4-ounce) cod filets, rinsed and patted dry
¼ teaspoon black pepper
⅛ teaspoon salt
2 tablespoons lemon juice

Topping

2½ tablespoons extra-virgin olive oil
1½ cup panko breadcrumbs
2 tablespoons grated Parmesan cheese
1 teaspoon dried dill
1 teaspoon grated lemon zest
¼ teaspoon salt
¼ cup chopped green onion

1 Preheat oven to 400°F.

2 Line a cookie sheet with foil. Lightly spray the foil with cooking spray. Arrange the fish filets in a single layer. Sprinkle evenly with black pepper and salt. Bake, uncovered, 10 minutes or until opaque in the center.

3 Meanwhile, heat the oil in a large nonstick skillet over medium heat. Add the breadcrumbs and cook 1–2 minutes or until golden, stirring constantly. Remove from the heat, and stir in the remaining topping ingredients. Set aside.

4 Place fillets on serving platter or four individual dinner plates. Squeeze the lemon juice evenly over the fish. Spoon equal amounts of the breadcrumb mixture on top of each. Sprinkle chopped onions on top.

EXCHANGES/CHOICES
3 lean meat, 1 fat

Calories	260	**Potassium**	490 mg
Calories from Fat	100	**Total Carbohydrate**	15 g
Total Fat	11 g	Dietary Fiber	1 g
Saturated Fat	2.5 g	Sugars	1 g
Trans Fat	0 g	**Protein**	24 g
Cholesterol	55 mg	**Phosphorus**	250 mg
Sodium	470 mg		

Cornmeal-Crusted Fish Strips with Creamy Honey Mustard Sauce

SERVES: 4 / **SERVING SIZE:** 3 ounces cooked fish and 1 tablespoon sauce

1 Preheat oven to 200°F.

2 Whisk together the buttermilk and egg whites in a medium bowl. Place the fish in the bowl and toss gently until well coated.

3 Stir together the flour, cornmeal, garlic powder, dill, and black pepper. Working with one strip at a time, lightly coat pieces with the cornmeal mixture and set aside on separate plate.

4 Heat 1 tablespoon of the oil in a large non-stick skillet over medium heat. Tilt skillet to coat bottom lightly. Add half of the fish strips and cook 6 minutes, turning midway. Place on a separate plate and place in oven to keep warm. Repeat with remaining fish.

5 Meanwhile, stir together the sauce ingredients in a small bowl.

6 Sprinkle fish with the ¼ teaspoon salt and serve with the sauce.

½ cup fat-free buttermilk
2 large egg whites
1 pound fish filets (such as tilapia), cut in 1-inch strips lengthwise, rinsed, and patted dry
⅓ cup yellow cornmeal
1 tablespoon white, whole-wheat, or all-purpose flour
½ teaspoon garlic powder
½ teaspoon dried dill
¼ teaspoon black pepper
2 tablespoons canola oil, divided use
¼ teaspoon salt

Sauce
3 tablespoons light mayonnaise
2 teaspoons honey
1 teaspoon Dijon mustard
⅛ teaspoon salt

COOK'S TIP: Cut larger fish strips in half, if desired, for easier handling.

EXCHANGES/CHOICES
1 starch, 3 lean meat, 1 fat

Calories	260	**Potassium**	420 mg
Calories from Fat	110	**Total Carbohydrate**	13 g
Total Fat	12 g	Dietary Fiber	1 g
Saturated Fat	1.5 g	Sugars	4 g
Trans Fat	0 g	**Protein**	26 g
Cholesterol	60 mg	**Phosphorus**	290 mg
Sodium	480 mg		

Cod with Avocado Corn Salsa Salad, PAGE 141

Cod with Avocado Corn Salsa Salad

SERVES: 4 / **SERVING SIZE:** 3 ounces cooked fish and ½ cup salsa

 1 Preheat grill or grill pan coated with cooking spray to medium-high heat.

2 Combine all salsa ingredients, except the avocado, in a medium bowl. Gently stir in the avocado and set aside.

3 Brush both sides of the fish fillets with oil and sprinkle evenly with the cumin, ¼ teaspoon of the salt, and black pepper. Cook 4 minutes on each side or until opaque in center. Serve with salsa alongside.

Salsa
- **1** cup grape tomatoes, quartered
- **1** cup frozen corn kernels, thawed
- **¼** cup chopped cilantro
- **¼** cup finely chopped red onion or jalapeño chili pepper
- **2** tablespoons lime juice
- **1** tablespoon extra-virgin olive oil
- **¼** teaspoon salt
- **1** ripe medium avocado, peeled, seeded, and chopped

Fish
- **4** (4-ounce) cod fillets, rinsed and patted dry
- **1** tablespoon extra-virgin olive oil
- **½** teaspoon ground cumin
- **¼** teaspoon salt
- Black pepper to taste

EXCHANGES/CHOICES
2 vegetable, 3 lean meat, 1 fat

Calories	270	**Potassium**	810 mg
Calories from Fat	120	**Total Carbohydrate**	15 g
Total Fat	14 g	Dietary Fiber	4 g
Saturated Fat	2 g	Sugars	2 g
Trans Fat	0 g	**Protein**	23 g
Cholesterol	50 mg	**Phosphorus**	280 mg
Sodium	360 mg		

Grilled Tuna Steaks and Minted Cucumber Bulgur

SERVES: 4 / **SERVING SIZE:** 3 ounces cooked tuna and ¾ cup bulgur mixture

Bulgur

1½	cups water
⅓	cup uncooked quick-cooking bulgur
1	cup diced tomato
¾	cup diced cucumber
¼	cup diced red onion or 1 medium garlic clove, minced
½	cup chopped fresh mint
1½	tablespoons extra-virgin olive oil
1	tablespoon lemon juice
1	tablespoon cider vinegar
½	teaspoon salt

Fish

¼	teaspoon salt
¼	teaspoon black pepper
⅛–¼	teaspoon dried pepper flakes
4	(4-ounce) tuna steaks, rinsed and patted dry

1. Bring the water to a boil in a small saucepan over high heat. Stir in the bulgur, reduce the heat to medium low, cover, and cook 10 minutes or until slightly firm. Drain in a fine-mesh sieve and run under cold water to cool quickly, shaking off excess liquid. Place in a medium bowl with the remaining bulgur ingredients and set aside.

2. Stir together the salt, black pepper, and pepper flakes in a small bowl. Place the tuna on a dinner plate and sprinkle the mixture evenly over both sides of the tuna. Let stand 5 minutes.

3. Heat a grill pan coated with cooking spray over high heat. Cook tuna 2 minutes on each side or until very pink in center (do not overcook). Serve the bulgur mixture alongside.

EXCHANGES/CHOICES

½ starch, 1 vegetable, 4 lean meat

Calories	230	**Potassium**	720 mg
Calories from Fat	50	**Total Carbohydrate**	13 g
Total Fat	6 g	Dietary Fiber	3 g
Saturated Fat	1 g	Sugars	2 g
Trans Fat	0 g	**Protein**	30 g
Cholesterol	45 mg	**Phosphorus**	370 mg
Sodium	360 mg		

COOK'S TIP 1: The juices from the bulgur mixture will season the tuna as well.

COOK'S TIP 2: It's important not to cook the tuna too long or it will become dry and tough.

Grilled Salmon, Grilled Veggie Quinoa

SERVES: 4 / **SERVING SIZE:** 3 ounces cooked salmon and ½ cup quinoa mixture

1. Preheat grill or grill pan to medium-high heat.

2. Lightly coat the onion and squash with cooking spray and cook 3 minutes on each side.

3. Meanwhile, bring water to a boil in a small saucepan over high heat, stir in the quinoa, reduce heat to medium-low, cover, and simmer 10 minutes or until done. Drain in fine-mesh sieve, place in a medium bowl, cover to keep warm, and set aside.

4. Combine ½ teaspoon of the thyme, garlic powder, black pepper, and ¼ teaspoon of the salt in a small bowl. Lightly coat the salmon with cooking spray and sprinkle the thyme mixture evenly over the top of the salmon. Turn the vegetables and place the salmon, skin side up, alongside the vegetables. Cook for 5 minutes. Turn salmon and vegetables and cook 4–5 minutes or until the salmon flakes easily when tested with a fork.

5. Coarsely chop the vegetables and stir into the quinoa with the remaining ½ teaspoon thyme, ¼ teaspoon salt, and the oil. Serve alongside the salmon.

1 medium onion (about 4 ounces), cut into ½-inch-thick rounds or slices
1 medium yellow squash, cut in half lengthwise
Cooking spray
1 cup water
¼ cup dry quinoa
1 teaspoon dried thyme leaves, divided use
½ teaspoon garlic powder
½ teaspoon black pepper
½ teaspoon salt, divided use
1 pound salmon filet, cut into 4 pieces
2 teaspoons extra-virgin olive oil

COOK'S TIP: For variation: substitute for the onion with 1 medium red bell pepper, cut in half. Substitute for the yellow squash with zucchini.

EXCHANGES/CHOICES
1 starch, 1 vegetable, 3 lean meat

Calories	250	**Potassium**	660 mg
Calories from Fat	80	**Total Carbohydrate**	15 g
Total Fat	9 g	Dietary Fiber	2 g
Saturated Fat	1.5 g	Sugars	5 g
Trans Fat	0 g	**Protein**	28 g
Cholesterol	60 mg	**Phosphorus**	375 mg
Sodium	290 mg		

Spicy Shrimp and Tomato Pasta Toss

SERVES: 4 / **SERVING SIZE:** 1 cup

6	cups water
2	ounces multigrain spaghetti noodles, broken in half
8	ounces peeled raw shrimp
2	cups small broccoli florets
4	ounces sweet grape tomatoes, quartered
1–2	medium jalapeño, halved lengthwise, seeded and thinly sliced
2	medium garlic cloves, minced
¼	cup chopped fresh basil
2	tablespoons extra-virgin olive oil
½	teaspoon salt

1 Bring the water to a boil in a large saucepan over high heat. Add the pasta, return to a boil, and cook 7 minutes. Add the shrimp and cook 2 minutes. Add the broccoli and cook 2–3 minutes or until the shrimp is opaque in center.

2 Meanwhile, in a medium bowl, combine the remaining ingredients. Drain the pasta mixture and add to the tomato mixture. Toss until well blended.

EXCHANGES/CHOICES

1 starch, 1½ lean meat, 1 fat

Calories	170	**Potassium**	270 mg
Calories from Fat	70	**Total Carbohydrate**	15 g
Total Fat	8 g	Dietary Fiber	2 g
Saturated Fat	1 g	Sugars	2 g
Trans Fat	0 g	**Protein**	11 g
Cholesterol	70 mg	**Phosphorus**	210 mg
Sodium	540 mg		

Scallops and Shallots on Snow Peas

SERVES: 4 / **SERVING SIZE:** ½ cup scallops and ⅓ cup peas

1. In a shallow pan, such as a pie pan, combine flour and paprika and toss to blend thoroughly.

2. Place scallops on several layers of paper towels and gently press to release liquid. Add the scallops to the flour mixture and toss to coat, shake off excess flour mixture, and set aside.

3. Place a large nonstick skillet over medium heat until hot. Melt the butter, tilt skillet to coat bottom evenly. Add scallops and cook 3 minutes, turn, sprinkle ⅛ teaspoon salt evenly over all, and cook 2 minutes longer or until opaque in center. Set aside on separate plate.

4. To pan residue in skillet, heat the oil over medium heat, cook the shallots 3–4 minutes or until beginning to be richly browned.

5. Meanwhile, place ⅓ cup of the water in a shallow microwave-safe pan, such as a glass pie pan, add the snow peas, cover and microwave on high 3–4 minutes or until tender-crisp.

6. Add the remaining ⅓ cup water to the shallots and stir to release any browned bits. Add the scallops and cook 1 minute or until liquid is thickened slightly, stirring gently.

7. Drain the snow peas, sprinkle with ⅛ teaspoon of the salt, and place equal amounts on each of four dinner plates. Spoon the scallop mixture on top, sprinkle with the remaining ⅛ teaspoon salt, and the parsley. Serve with the lemon wedges.

3	tablespoons all-purpose flour
½	teaspoon paprika
1	pound scallops, rinsed and patted dry
2	tablespoons light butter
⅜	teaspoon salt, divided use
½	cup finely chopped shallots or yellow onion
⅔	cup water, divided use
1	teaspoon extra-virgin olive oil
6	ounces snow peas, stemmed
2	tablespoons finely chopped Italian parsley or cilantro
1	medium lemon, quartered

EXCHANGES/CHOICES
1 starch, 2 lean meat

Calories	190	**Potassium**	560 mg
Calories from Fat	45	**Total Carbohydrate**	15 g
Total Fat	5 g	Dietary Fiber	3 g
Saturated Fat	1 g	Sugars	4 g
Trans Fat	0 g	**Protein**	22 g
Cholesterol	25 mg	**Phosphorus**	320 mg
Sodium	400 mg		

Beef Sirloin with Shallot-Mushroom Sauce

SERVES: 4 / **SERVING SIZE:** 3 ounces cooked beef and ½ cup mushroom sauce

1   tablespoon canola oil, divided use
1   cup thinly sliced shallots (about 4 medium)
1   pound boneless beef sirloin, trimmed of fat
½   teaspoon salt, divided use
¼   teaspoon black pepper
1   pound sliced mushrooms
½   cup dry red wine
1½ to 2   tablespoons balsamic vinegar
2   teaspoons Worcestershire sauce
1   teaspoon sugar
1   tablespoon diet margarine, such as Smart Balance
2   tablespoons finely chopped parsley (optional)

1 Heat 1 teaspoon of the oil in a large non-stick skillet over medium-high heat. Add the shallots and cook 5 minutes or until richly browned, stirring occasionally. Set aside on separate plate.

2 Heat 1 teaspoon of the oil in the skillet. Sprinkle both sides of the beef with ¼ teaspoon of the salt and pepper. Cook the beef 4 minutes on each side. Place on cutting board. Let stand 3 minutes before slicing against the grain.

3 Meanwhile, add the remaining 1 teaspoon oil to the pan residue in the skillet. Cook the mushrooms 4 minutes, stirring occasionally. Stir in the wine, vinegar, Worcestershire sauce, sugar, and remaining ¼ teaspoon salt. Bring to a boil over medium-high heat, cook 7 minutes or until thickened. Add the shallots and diet margarine and cook 1 minute. Serve over the beef slices and sprinkle with additional black pepper and parsley, if desired.

EXCHANGES/CHOICES

½ starch, 1 vegetable, 4 lean meat

Calories	260	**Potassium**	990 mg
Calories from Fat	90	**Total Carbohydrate**	14 g
Total Fat	10 g	Dietary Fiber	3 g
Saturated Fat	2 g	Sugars	8 g
Trans Fat	0 g	**Protein**	31 g
Cholesterol	75 mg	**Phosphorus**	380 mg
Sodium	340 mg		

COOK'S TIP: The heat from the sauce will reheat the beef slices.

Beef Kabobs with Potatoes and Soy Balsamic Sauce

SERVES: 4 / **SERVING SIZE:** 1 kabob plus about 1 tablespoon sauce

1. In a small bowl, whisk together the sauce ingredients. Place the beef in a quart-size resealable plastic bag, add 2 tablespoons of the sauce, seal tightly, and toss back and forth until well coated. Refrigerate beef and remaining sauce (in a separate container) overnight or at least 2 hours, turning occasionally.

2. Preheat the grill or grill pan on medium-high.

3. Place the potatoes and ¼ cup water in a medium microwave-safe bowl, cover with plastic wrap, and microwave on high for 5 minutes or until just tender when pierced with a fork. Drain in a colander and run under cold water to stop cooking process.

4. Remove beef and discard remaining soy sauce mixture in the bag. Alternately thread beef with the vegetables onto skewers. Cook 4 minutes on each side or to desired doneness.

5. Meanwhile, place the reserved sauce in the microwave for 1 minute or until heated.

6. Place skewers on each of four dinner plates and serve the sauce alongside or equal amounts spooned over each serving (about 1 tablespoon per serving).

Sauce
- 2½ tablespoons light soy sauce
- 2½ tablespoons balsamic vinegar
- 1 tablespoon extra-virgin olive oil
- 2 teaspoons Worcestershire sauce
- 2 teaspoons water
- 1 teaspoon dried oregano leaves

Kabobs
- 1 pound boneless sirloin, trimmed and cut into 16 cubes
- 8 ounces small new potatoes (about 4), scrubbed and quartered
- ¼ cup water
- 1 medium red bell pepper, cut into 16 pieces
- ½ large red onion, cut into 4 wedges, layers separated (4 ounces total)
- 8 (12-inch) bamboo or metal skewers

COOK'S TIP: Sirloin can be very tough if cooked too long; it's best to cook until very pink in center.

EXCHANGES/CHOICES
1 starch, 3½ lean meat

Calories	240		**Potassium**	690 mg
Calories from Fat	40		**Total Carbohydrate**	15 g
Total Fat	6 g		Dietary Fiber	1 g
Saturated Fat	1.5 g		Sugars	5 g
Trans Fat	0 g		**Protein**	27 g
Cholesterol	70 mg		**Phosphorus**	280 mg
Sodium	480 mg			

Sweet Home Beef and Veggie Pot Roast, PAGE 149

Sweet Home Beef and Veggie Pot Roast

SERVES: 4 / **SERVING SIZE:** about 3½ oz beef, ¾ cup vegetables, and 2 tablespoons sauce

1 Coat a 3½–4 quart slow cooker with cooking spray. Place the carrots, onion, and celery in bottom of the slow cooker. Top with the beef. Spoon the water, vinegar, and Worcestershire over the beef. Sprinkle evenly with black pepper and onion soup mix. Cover and cook on high setting for 4 hours or on low setting for 8 hours.

Cooking spray
4 medium carrots, scrubbed, halved lengthwise, and cut into 3-inch pieces
1 medium onion (4 ounces), cut in eighths
2 medium celery stalks, halved lengthwise and cut into 3-inch pieces
1¼ pounds boneless lean chuck roast, trimmed of fat
2 tablespoons water
1 tablespoon balsamic vinegar
2 teaspoons Worcestershire sauce
½ teaspoon black pepper
1 ounce packet dried onion soup mix

COOK'S TIP: When buying chuck roast, purchase 4 ounces or more than the required amount in ingredient list, because there is "hidden" fat that may need to be trimmed on the underside of the beef or throughout beef. The weight given in the ingredient list is the weight AFTER it has been trimmed of fat.

EXCHANGES/CHOICES
½ starch, 1 vegetable, 4 lean meat

Calories	250	**Potassium**	800 mg
Calories from Fat	50	**Total Carbohydrate**	15 g
Total Fat	6 g	Dietary Fiber	3 g
Saturated Fat	2 g	Sugars	6 g
Trans Fat	0 g	**Protein**	33 g
Cholesterol	90 mg	**Phosphorus**	330 mg
Sodium	506 mg		

Italian Veggie Smothered Beef Patties

SERVES: 4 / **SERVING SIZE:** 3 ounces cooked beef and 1 cup vegetable mixture

1	pound extra lean ground beef
2	teaspoons canola oil, divided use
1	cup diced yellow onion
4	ounces sliced mushrooms
1½	cups chopped green or yellow bell pepper
1	medium zucchini (6 ounces), trimmed and sliced
1	(14.5-ounce) can no-salt-added stewed tomatoes
2	teaspoons dried basil leaves
2	teaspoons balsamic vinegar
½	teaspoon salt
2	ounces fat-free feta, crumbled

1 Shape ground beef into 4 patties. Heat a large nonstick skillet with 1 teaspoon of the oil over medium-high heat. Sprinkle with ¼ teaspoon of the salt. Cook patties 3 minutes on each side or until slightly pink in center. Set aside on separate plate.

2 Heat the remaining 1 teaspoon oil over medium-high heat and cook the onions for 3 minutes or until translucent. Add the mushrooms, peppers, zucchini, and tomatoes. Bring to a boil over medium-high heat, reduce to medium, and cook, uncovered, 8 minutes or until slightly thickened and peppers are just tender-crisp.

3 Stir in the basil, vinegar, and salt, add the patties and any accumulated juices, spoon some of the tomato mixture over the patties, and cook 1 minute to heat through and cook patties slightly. Remove from heat and sprinkle with the feta, cover, and let stand 3 minutes to allow flavors to blend.

EXCHANGES/CHOICES
3 vegetable, 4 lean meat

Calories	260	**Potassium**	960 mg	
Calories from Fat	70	**Total Carbohydrate**	14 g	
Total Fat	8 g	Dietary Fiber	4 g	
Saturated Fat	2.8 g	Sugars	9 g	
Trans Fat	0 g	**Protein**	29 g	
Cholesterol	70 mg	**Phosphorus**	340 mg	
Sodium	460 mg			

COOK'S TIP: To make this easy dish even easier, pick up pre-cut vegetables in the produce aisle in major supermarkets.

Blue Cheese Beef and Noodle Toss

SERVES: 4 / **SERVING SIZE:** 1⅓ cups

 1 Cook pasta according to package directions, omitting any salt or fat.

Meanwhile, heat a large skillet over medium-high heat. Cook the beef and onions 4 minutes, stirring frequently. Stir in the mushrooms and cook 8 minutes or until mushrooms are beginning to brown. Add the tomatoes, cook 2 minutes or until just beginning to soften. Remove from heat.

2 Stir in the drained pasta, ¼ cup water, basil, salt, and black pepper. Sprinkle with the cheese.

2	ounces uncooked no-yolk egg noodles
1	pound extra-lean ground beef
¼	cup diced onion
8	ounces whole mushrooms, wiped clean with a damp cloth and quartered
¾	cup grape tomatoes, quartered
¼	cup water
2	tablespoons chopped fresh basil or 2 teaspoons dried basil
½	teaspoon salt
¼	teaspoon black pepper
½	ounce reduced-fat blue cheese, crumbled

EXCHANGES/CHOICES
1 starch, 4 lean meat

Calories	250	**Potassium**	720 mg
Calories from Fat	70	**Total Carbohydrate**	14 g
Total Fat	8 g	Dietary Fiber	2 g
Saturated Fat	3.6 g	Sugars	3 g
Trans Fat	0 g	**Protein**	30 g
Cholesterol	90 mg	**Phosphorus**	340 mg
Sodium	380 mg		

Pork Tenderloin with Pineapple-Horseradish Sauce

SERVES: 4 / **SERVING SIZE:** 3 ounces cooked pork and 3 tablespoons pineapple mixture

- **1** pound pork tenderloin
- **1** teaspoon ground cumin
- **½** teaspoon black pepper
- **¼** teaspoon salt
- **1** teaspoon canola oil
- **3** tablespoons apricot fruit spread
- **1** (8-ounce) can crushed pineapple in its own juice, drained
- **1** tablespoon prepared horseradish

1 Preheat the oven to 425°F.

2 In a small bowl, combine the cumin, pepper, and salt and sprinkle evenly over the pork. Heat the oil in a medium nonstick skillet over medium-high heat. Brown the pork 2 minutes on each side. Coat an 11 × 7-inch baking dish with cooking spray. Place the pork in the baking dish. Bake 15–18 minutes or until internal temperature reaches 145°F. Place on cutting board and let stand 5 minutes before thinly slicing.

3 Meanwhile, place the fruit spread in a small microwave-safe bowl. Microwave on high for 30 seconds or until melted. Stir in the pineapple and the horseradish. Let cool completely. Serve with the pork.

EXCHANGES/CHOICES
1 fruit, 3 lean meat

Calories	200	**Potassium**	680 mg
Calories from Fat	45	**Total Carbohydrate**	15 g
Total Fat	5 g	Dietary Fiber	0 g
Saturated Fat	1.5 g	Sugars	12 g
Trans Fat	0 g	**Protein**	23 g
Cholesterol	60 mg	**Phosphorus**	330 mg
Sodium	390 mg		

Pork Tenderloin with Chipotle-Orange Veggies

SERVES: 4 / **SERVING SIZE:** ¾ cup vegetable mixture and 3 ounces cooked pork

1. Preheat oven to 425°F.

2. Place the onions, peppers, and squash in a 13 × 9-inch dish, toss with 1 tablespoon of the oil, and arrange in a single layer on bottom.

3. Season all sides of pork with the garlic powder, salt, and black pepper. Heat the remaining 1 teaspoon oil in a large skillet over medium-high heat. Brown the pork on all sides, about 6 minutes total. Place in the baking dish nestled into the veggies.

4. Pour the orange juice and salsa into the skillet with the pan residue. Bring to a boil over medium-high heat and continue boiling 5 minutes or until thickened slightly. Pour evenly over the pork and veggies.

5. Bake, uncovered, 20 minutes or until pork reaches 145°F when insert with a meat thermometer. Remove the pork and place on cutting board. Let stand 5 minutes before thinly slicing. Meanwhile, return the vegetables to the oven and continue to cook 8–10 minutes or until squash is tender. Serve pork with the vegetable mixture.

1	cup chopped onion
1	large red bell pepper, chopped
1	medium yellow squash, quartered lengthwise and chopped
1	tablespoon plus 1 teaspoon canola oil, divided use
1	pound pork tenderloin
½	teaspoon garlic powder
¼	teaspoon salt
¼	teaspoon black pepper
¾	cup orange juice
½	cup chipotle salsa

EXCHANGES/CHOICES
3 vegetable, 3 lean meat

Calories	230	**Potassium**	840 mg
Calories from Fat	60	**Total Carbohydrate**	14 g
Total Fat	7 g	Dietary Fiber	2 g
Saturated Fat	1 g	Sugars	9 g
Trans Fat	0 g	**Protein**	26 g
Cholesterol	70 mg	**Phosphorus**	330 mg
Sodium	390 mg		

Pork Chops with Broccoli Almond Rice

SERVES: 4 / **SERVING SIZE:** 3 ounces cooked pork plus about ½ cup rice mixture

1	ounce slivered almonds
1	tablespoon canola oil
4	boneless pork chops (1 pound total), trimmed of fat
¼	teaspoon salt and ⅛ teaspoon salt, divided use
1	teaspoon chili powder
¾	cup water
1	cup small broccoli florets
1	cup frozen cooked brown rice
1–2	teaspoons hot sauce, such as Sriracha
1½	teaspoons light soy sauce

1. Heat a large skillet over medium heat. Add the almonds and cook 2 minutes or until lightly browned, stirring frequently, and set aside. Heat oil and season pork with ⅛ teaspoon salt and chili powder. Cook 4 minutes on each side or until barely pink in center and set aside. To pan residue, add the water, broccoli, and rice, reduce heat, cover, and cook on medium-low for 3 minutes or until broccoli is tender-crisp. Stir in the almonds and remaining ¼ teaspoon salt. Top with the pork chops and any accumulated juices. In a small bowl, combine the hot sauce and soy sauce and drizzle evenly over all. Cover and cook 1 minute on medium low to heat pork chops.

EXCHANGES/CHOICES
1 starch, 3 lean meat, 1 fat

Calories	270	**Potassium**	570 mg
Calories from Fat	110	**Total Carbohydrate**	15 g
Total Fat	12 g	Dietary Fiber	2 g
Saturated Fat	2 g	Sugars	1 g
Trans Fat	0 g	**Protein**	27 g
Cholesterol	70 mg	**Phosphorus**	360 mg
Sodium	380 mg		

COOK'S TIP: Be sure to cut the broccoli florets into small pieces for better distribution and quick cooking.

Grilled Pork and Sweet Potato Kabobs

SERVES: 4 / **SERVING SIZE:** 1 skewer

 1 Preheat grill or grill pan to medium-high heat.

2 Place the sweet potatoes and water in a shallow microwavable pan, such as a pie pan, cover, and microwave on high setting for 3–4 minutes or until potatoes are just tender, stirring midway (do not overcook). Drain sweet potatoes; rinse with cold water.

3 On each of four 10- to 12-inch skewers, starting and end, with the pork, carefully thread pork, sweet potatoes, and zucchini (with cut side facing out) alternately, leaving ¼-inch space between each piece. Grill for 10–12 minutes, uncovered, or until pork is barely pink in center.

4 Meanwhile, in a small bowl, whisk together the mustard, oil, and jam.

5 Remove the skewers from the grill, sprinkle with the salt and pepper, and brush the mustard mixture evenly over all.

8	ounces sweet potatoes, peeled and cut into 8 pieces
¼	cup water
12	ounces pork tenderloin, cut into 12 pieces
1	small zucchini, cut into 8 rounds
½	large red bell pepper, cut into 8 cubes
¼	teaspoon salt
¼	teaspoon black pepper
2	tablespoons coarse-ground Dijon mustard
1	tablespoon extra-virgin olive oil
1	tablespoon sugar-free raspberry jam

EXCHANGES/CHOICES
1 starch, 2½ lean meat

Calories	190	**Potassium**	800 mg
Calories from Fat	45	**Total Carbohydrate**	15 g
Total Fat	5 g	Dietary Fiber	3 g
Saturated Fat	1 g	Sugars	4 g
Trans Fat	0 g	**Protein**	19 g
Cholesterol	40 mg	**Phosphorus**	300 mg
Sodium	520 mg		

Sides

VEGETABLES

Acorn Squash with Delicate Almond Sauce
Hearty Skillet Kale
Herbed Panko Asparagus Spears
Parmesan Garlic Spinach
Baked Tomatoes with Panko and Parmesan

GRAINS

Bulgur and Browned Onions with Apricots
Sauteed Artichoke-Garlic Penne
Spicy Cheddar Broccoli Rice
Grilled Corn with Buttery Parsley
Sweet Cumin Corn, Red Pepper, and Carrots
Rosemary Garlic Multi-Grain Bread

POTATOES

Sneaky Mashed Potatoes

Lemon Tarragon Veggie Potato Toss

Sauteed Mushroom and Onion Skillet
Potatoes

Green Bean-New Potato Roast

Roasted Cauliflower, Onions, and Sweet
Potatoes

Brown Sugar Sweet Potato and Carrots

LEGUMES

Lentils, Carrots, and Ginger

Black Beans and Tomatoes with Lime

Sweet Peas with Mint and Green Onion

Acorn Squash with Delicate Almond Sauce

SERVES: 4 / **SERVING SIZE:** 1 squash quarter and 2 tablespoons sauce

1	pound acorn squash, pierced in several areas with a fork
¼	cup water
1	ounce sliced almonds, toasted
½	teaspoon almond extract
4	teaspoons diet margarine, such as Smart Balance
2	tablespoons sugar-free maple or pancake syrup
¼	teaspoon salt

1 Place the squash in the microwave on high setting for 3 minutes. Remove from the microwave and cut in quarters. Using a spoon, scrape the seeds and connecting membrane from the center of each piece.

2 Place the squash in a shallow microwave-safe pan, such as a glass pie pan. Pour the water in the pan. Cover with plastic wrap and microwave on high for 9–10 minutes or until squash is tender when pierced with a fork.

3 Place the squash pieces cut side up on individual dinner plates. Top each with equal amounts of the almonds. To pan residue, add the remaining ingredients and microwave on high 1 minute or until margarine has melted. Whisk until well blended and spoon over the almonds.

EXCHANGES/CHOICES
1 starch, 1 fat

Calories	120	**Potassium**	440 mg
Calories from Fat	45	**Total Carbohydrate**	15 g
Total Fat	5 g	Dietary Fiber	3 g
Saturated Fat	1 g	Sugars	0 g
Trans Fat	0 g	**Protein**	3 g
Cholesterol	0 mg	**Phosphorus**	75 mg
Sodium	140 mg		

Hearty Skillet Kale

SERVES: 4 / **SERVING SIZE:** About a scant cup

1 Heat 1 teaspoon of the oil in a large non-stick skillet over medium-high heat. Add the onions and cook 2 minutes, stirring frequently. Add the garlic and cook 15 seconds, stirring constantly. Add half of the kale and cook 2 minutes or until just beginning to wilt, stirring gently using two utensils as you would a stir-fry. Add the remaining kale and remaining ingredients, except the lemon or vinegar, and cook 5–6 minutes or until wilted, stirring frequently. Sprinkle the lemon or vinegar evenly over all.

1½ tablespoons extra-virgin olive oil, divided use
½ cup diced onion
2 garlic cloves, minced
1 pound kale, ribs removed, leaves roughly chopped
1 teaspoon sugar
½ teaspoon salt
¼ teaspoon freshly ground black pepper
⅛–¼ teaspoon red pepper flakes
2 tablespoons fresh lemon juice or cider vinegar

EXCHANGES/CHOICES
3 vegetable, 1 fat

Calories	120	**Potassium**	600 mg
Calories from Fat	50	**Total Carbohydrate**	14 g
Total Fat	6 g	Dietary Fiber	3 g
Saturated Fat	1 g	Sugars	5 g
Trans Fat	0 g	**Protein**	5 g
Cholesterol	0 mg	**Phosphorus**	110 mg
Sodium	240 mg		

Herbed Panko Asparagus Spears, PAGE 163

Herbed Panko Asparagus Spears

SERVES: 4 / **SERVING SIZE:** 6 asparagus spears, 2 tablespoons sauce, and 2 tablespoons crumbs

1   Heat the oil in a large skillet over medium-high heat. Add the breadcrumbs and cook 1–2 minutes or until golden, stirring constantly. Set aside on separate plate.

2   Bring the water to a boil in the skillet over medium-high heat. Add the asparagus, return to a boil, reduce heat, cover, and simmer 3 minutes or until just tender. Drain well, discarding water. Place the asparagus on a serving plate.

3   Meanwhile, in a small bowl, whisk together the sour cream, mayonnaise, milk, mustard, tarragon, and salt. Place in the skillet over medium-low heat and cook 1 minute or until heated, stirring constantly. Spoon over the asparagus and sprinkle with the breadcrumbs.

2	teaspoons extra-virgin olive oil
1/3	cup panko breadcrumbs
1	cup water
1	pound asparagus spears, trimmed
1/4	cup fat-free sour cream
3	tablespoons light mayonnaise
2	tablespoons fat-free milk
1 1/2	teaspoons prepared mustard
1/4	teaspoon dried tarragon leaves
1/4	teaspoon salt

EXCHANGES/CHOICES
3 vegetable, 1 fat

Calories	120	**Potassium**	290 mg
Calories from Fat	45	**Total Carbohydrate**	15 g
Total Fat	5 g	Dietary Fiber	3 g
Saturated Fat	1 g	Sugars	4 g
Trans Fat	0 g	**Protein**	5 g
Cholesterol	<5 mg	**Phosphorus**	100 mg
Sodium	300 mg		

Parmesan Garlic Spinach

SERVES: 4 / **SERVING SIZE:** ¾ cup

1	teaspoon canola oil
16	ounces fresh baby spinach
2	tablespoons reduced-fat cream cheese (tub style)
1	tablespoon diet margarine
1	medium garlic clove, minced
1	tablespoon grated Parmesan cheese

1 Heat the oil in a large nonstick skillet over medium-high heat. Add half of the spinach and cook 1 minute or until *just* beginning to wilt slightly, gently tossing using two utensils, as you would a stir-fry. Add the remaining spinach and garlic to the spinach in the skillet and cook 1 minute, or until just wilted, tossing gently and constantly.

2 Remove from heat, stir in the remaining ingredients, except the Parmesan. Toss gently until cream cheese has just melted. Sprinkle evenly with the cheese. Serve immediately for peak flavors.

EXCHANGES/CHOICES
1 vegetable, 1 fat

Calories	80	**Potassium**	660 mg
Calories from Fat	25	**Total Carbohydrate**	13 g
Total Fat	3 g	Dietary Fiber	5 g
Saturated Fat	1.5 g	Sugars	1 g
Trans Fat	0 g	**Protein**	4 g
Cholesterol	5 mg	**Phosphorus**	75 mg
Sodium	270 mg		

COOK'S TIP: The amount of spinach seems to "take over" the skillet, but just give it 1 minute and see it subside!

Baked Tomatoes with Panko and Parmesan

SERVES: 4 / **SERVING SIZE:** 2 tomato halves

1 Preheat oven 350°F.

2 Coat a nonstick baking sheet with cooking spray, arrange tomato halves on bottom of pan, drizzle vinegar evenly over all.

3 In a small bowl, combine the remaining ingredients, except Parmesan. Toss gently and spoon equal amounts over each tomato.

4 Bake 20 minutes or until tomatoes are tender and crumb topping is beginning to brown. Remove from oven and sprinkle with Parmesan cheese. Let stand 5 minutes to absorb flavors.

Cooking spray
4 large tomatoes (about 6 ounces each), halved crosswise
1 tablespoon cider vinegar
2 teaspoons dried basil leaves
½ teaspoon salt
½ cup panko breadcrumbs
2 tablespoons canola oil
2 tablespoons grated Parmesan cheese

EXCHANGES/CHOICES
½ starch, 1 vegetable, 1½ fat

Calories	130	**Potassium**	420 mg
Calories from Fat	70	**Total Carbohydrate**	12 g
Total Fat	8 g	Dietary Fiber	2 g
Saturated Fat	1 g	Sugars	5 g
Trans Fat	0 g	**Protein**	3 g
Cholesterol	<5 mg	**Phosphorus**	60 mg
Sodium	270 mg		

Bulgur and Browned Onions with Apricots

SERVES: 4 / **SERVING SIZE:** ½ cup

¾	cup water
⅓	cup quick-cooking bulgur
1	teaspoon canola oil
⅔	cup diced onions
1½	ounces chopped walnuts, toasted (⅓ cup)
4	dried apricot halves, cut in thin slices
¾	teaspoon curry powder
¼	teaspoon ground cumin
¼	teaspoon salt
⅛	teaspoon dried pepper flakes

 In a small saucepan, bring water to boil over high heat, stir in the bulgur, reduce heat, cover tightly, and simmer 12 minutes or until just tender.

 Meanwhile, heat the oil in a medium non-stick skillet over medium-high heat. Tilt skillet to coat lightly and cook the onions 6 minutes or until richly browned, stirring frequently. Remove from heat.

 Drain bulgur, if necessary, in a fine mesh strainer, shaking off excess liquid. Stir into the onions with the remaining ingredients.

EXCHANGES/CHOICES
1 starch, 1½ fat

Calories	140	**Potassium**	190 mg
Calories from Fat	70	**Total Carbohydrate**	15 g
Total Fat	8 g	Dietary Fiber	4 g
Saturated Fat	0.5 g	Sugars	4 g
Trans Fat	0 g	**Protein**	3 g
Cholesterol	0 mg	**Phosphorus**	80 mg
Sodium	105 mg		

Sauteed Artichoke-Garlic Penne

SERVES: 4 / **SERVING SIZE:** ¾ cup

1. Cook the pasta according to package directions, omitting any salt or fat. Drain well.

2. Heat the oil in a medium nonstick skillet over medium-high heat. Add the artichokes, reduce the heat to medium, and cook 4 minutes or until lightly golden, stirring occasionally. Add the pasta and garlic and cook 1 minute, stirring gently. Remove from heat, stir in the salt.

2 ounces uncooked multigrain penne pasta
1 tablespoon extra-virgin olive oil
1 (14-ounce) can quartered artichoke hearts, drained and patted dry on paper towels
2 medium garlic cloves, minced
¼ teaspoon salt

COOK'S TIP: It's very important to make sure that the artichoke hearts are patted dry or they will "spatter" and won't lightly brown.

EXCHANGES/CHOICES
1 starch, 1 vegetable, 1 fat

Calories	110	**Potassium**	320 mg
Calories from Fat	40	**Total Carbohydrate**	14 g
Total Fat	4 g	Dietary Fiber	1 g
Saturated Fat	0 g	Sugars	1 g
Trans Fat	0 g	**Protein**	4 g
Cholesterol	0 mg	**Phosphorus**	110 mg
Sodium	260 mg		

Spicy Cheddar Broccoli Rice

SERVES: 4 / **SERVING SIZE:** ½ cup

1	teaspoon canola oil
¼	cup diced onions
1	medium jalapeño, finely chopped and seeded, if desired
1½	cups small broccoli florets
1	cup frozen brown rice
½	cup water
1	ounce reduced-fat sharp cheddar cheese
¼	teaspoon salt

1 Heat the oil in a medium nonstick skillet over medium heat. Cook the onion and jalapeño 4 minutes or until translucent. Add the rice, broccoli, and water. Bring to a boil over medium-high heat. Reduce heat to medium low, cover, and simmer 7–8 minutes or until rice is tender. Remove from heat.

2 Gently stir in the cheese and salt.

EXCHANGES/CHOICES
½ starch, 1 vegetable, ½ fat

Calories	100	**Potassium**	190 mg
Calories from Fat	30	**Total Carbohydrate**	15 g
Total Fat	3 g	Dietary Fiber	2 g
Saturated Fat	1 g	Sugars	2 g
Trans Fat	0 g	**Protein**	3 g
Cholesterol	<5 mg	**Phosphorus**	120 mg
Sodium	230 mg		

Grilled Corn with Buttery Parsley

SERVES: 4 / **SERVING SIZE:** 1 ear of corn and 1½ teaspoons margarine mixture

1 Coat ears of corn with cooking spray, wrap each in a sheet of foil, diagonally, and twist the ends.

2 Heat a grill or grill pan over medium-high heat until hot. Cook corn 20 minutes or until tender and beginning to brown, turning frequently.

3 Meanwhile, in a small bowl, stir together the remaining ingredients. Unwrap the corn and spread equal amounts of the margarine mixture over all.

4	small ears corn on the cob, husks and silks removed
	Cooking spray
4	(12-inch) sheets of foil
4	teaspoons diet margarine, such as Smart Balance
¼	teaspoon dried thyme leaves
2	teaspoons finely chopped fresh parsley
¼	teaspoon salt
⅛	teaspoon black pepper

EXCHANGES/CHOICES
1 starch, ½ fat

Calories	80	**Potassium**	250 mg
Calories from Fat	20	**Total Carbohydrate**	14 g
Total Fat	2.5 g	Dietary Fiber	2 g
Saturated Fat	1 g	Sugars	2 g
Trans Fat	0 g	**Protein**	2 g
Cholesterol	0 mg	**Phosphorus**	80 mg
Sodium	190 mg		

Sweet Cumin Corn, Red Pepper, and Carrots

SERVES: 4 / **SERVING SIZE:** ½ cup

1	tablespoon canola oil
1	cup diced carrots
1	cup frozen corn kernels
½	cup diced red bell pepper
½	teaspoon ground cumin
1	teaspoon sugar
¼	teaspoon salt
⅛	teaspoon cayenne pepper

 Heat the oil in a medium nonstick skillet over medium-high heat. Add the carrots, stir until well coated, reduce heat to medium, cover, and cook 5 minutes or until just tender and beginning to lightly brown.

2. Stir in the remaining ingredients, cook 1–2 minutes to heat through.

EXCHANGES/CHOICES
½ starch, 1 vegetable, 1 fat

Calories	90	**Potassium**	230 mg
Calories from Fat	40	**Total Carbohydrate**	14 g
Total Fat	4 g	Dietary Fiber	2 g
Saturated Fat	0.5 g	Sugars	4 g
Trans Fat	0 g	**Protein**	2 g
Cholesterol	0 mg	**Phosphorus**	45 mg
Sodium	125 mg		

Rosemary Garlic Multi-Grain Bread

SERVES: 4 / **SERVING SIZE:** 2 slices

 1 Preheat broiler.

2 Using a serrated knife, carefully cut the bread into 8 thin slices. Place on a baking sheet and broil 1 minute, turn, and broil 30 seconds or until lightly toasted. Watch closely so it doesn't burn. Remove from broiler. Let stand 5 minutes to harden slightly.

3 Heat 1 teaspoon of the oil in a small skillet over medium heat. Cook the onion 2–3 minutes or until just beginning to turn golden. Add the garlic, parsley, and rosemary. Cook 15 seconds. Remove from heat. Stir in the remaining oil. Spoon or brush equal amounts on each bread slice. Sprinkle with cheese.

4 ounces whole-grain Italian bread
2 tablespoons extra-virgin olive oil, divided use
¼ cup finely chopped red onion
2 medium garlic cloves, minced
2 tablespoons finely chopped parsley
1½ teaspoons chopped fresh rosemary or ½ teaspoon dried rosemary
4 teaspoons grated Parmesan cheese

COOK'S TIP: The parsley mixture will be thick, but is packed with high flavored ingredients . . . a little goes a long way!

EXCHANGES/CHOICES
1 starch, 2 fat

Calories	150	**Potassium**	100 mg
Calories from Fat	80	**Total Carbohydrate**	14 g
Total Fat	9 g	Dietary Fiber	2 g
Saturated Fat	1.5 g	Sugars	2 g
Trans Fat	0 g	**Protein**	5 g
Cholesterol	<5 mg	**Phosphorus**	80 mg
Sodium	150 mg		

Sneaky Mashed Potatoes

SERVES: 4 / **SERVING SIZE:** ½ cup

4	cups water
8	ounces Yukon Gold or red potatoes, peeled, if desired, and chopped
12	ounces fresh or frozen cauliflower florets
3	tablespoons fat-free milk
¼	cup diet margarine (such as Smart Balance)
¼ to ½	teaspoon dried thyme leaves
¼ to ½	teaspoon garlic powder
½	teaspoon salt
¼	teaspoon black pepper

1. Bring water to a boil in a large saucepan over high heat. Add the potatoes and cauliflower, return to a boil, reduce heat, cover, and simmer 7 minutes or until vegetables are tender. Drain well, shaking off excess liquid.

2. Place the vegetables in a blender with the remaining ingredients. Purée until smooth.

EXCHANGES/CHOICES
1 starch, 1 fat

Calories	110	**Potassium**	540 mg
Calories from Fat	45	**Total Carbohydrate**	15 g
Total Fat	5 g	Dietary Fiber	3 g
Saturated Fat	1.5 g	Sugars	3 g
Trans Fat	0 g	**Protein**	3 g
Cholesterol	<5 mg	**Phosphorus**	90 mg
Sodium	330 mg		

Lemon Tarragon Veggie Potato Toss

1. Heat the oil in a large nonstick skillet over medium-high heat. Stir in the potatoes, bell pepper, and onions. Reduce heat to medium, cover, and cook 8–10 minutes or until potatoes are tender, stirring occasionally. Remove from heat.

2. Gently stir in the remaining ingredients. Cover and let stand 5 minutes to absorb flavors.

1	tablespoon extra-virgin olive oil
10	ounces new potatoes, cut into ½-inch wedges
1	cup diced green bell pepper
½	cup diced onions
1½	teaspoons chopped fresh tarragon or ½ teaspoon dried tarragon leaves
1	teaspoon grated lemon zest
½	teaspoon salt
⅛	teaspoon black pepper

EXCHANGES/CHOICES
1 starch, ½ fat

Calories	100	**Potassium**	330 mg
Calories from Fat	40	**Total Carbohydrate**	15 g
Total Fat	4 g	Dietary Fiber	1 g
Saturated Fat	0.5 g	Sugars	3 g
Trans Fat	0 g	**Protein**	2 g
Cholesterol	25 mg	**Phosphorus**	40 mg
Sodium	260 mg		

Sauteed Mushroom and Onion Skillet Potatoes

SERVES: 4/ **SERVING SIZE:** ¾ cup

1 tablespoon extra-virgin olive oil (divided use)
1 cup diced onions
8 ounces whole mushrooms, wiped with a damp cloth and quartered
8 ounces red potatoes, diced
1 medium garlic clove, minced
⅛ teaspoon black pepper
½ teaspoon salt

1 Heat 1 teaspoon of the oil in a large non-stick skillet over medium-high heat. Cook the onions 4 minutes or until edges are beginning to brown, stirring occasionally. Add 1 teaspoon of the oil, cook the mushrooms 3 minutes or until beginning to release their juices. Add the remaining 1 teaspoon oil, potatoes, garlic, and pepper.

2 Reduce the heat to medium low, cover, and cook 10 minutes or until potatoes are tender, stirring occasionally. Remove from heat.

3 Stir in the salt, cover, and let stand 5–10 minutes to absorb flavors.

EXCHANGES/CHOICES
1 starch, ½ fat

Calories	100	**Potassium**	500 mg
Calories from Fat	40	**Total Carbohydrate**	15 g
Total Fat	4 g	Dietary Fiber	2 g
Saturated Fat	0.5 g	Sugars	4 g
Trans Fat	0 g	**Protein**	3 g
Cholesterol	0 mg	**Phosphorus**	100 mg
Sodium	210 mg		

Green Bean–New Potato Roast

SERVES: 4 / **SERVING SIZE:** 1 cup

 Preheat the oven to 425°F.

2 Place the green beans and potatoes on large foil-lined baking sheet. Drizzle with the oil and toss gently until well coated. Arrange vegetables in a single layer and bake 10 minutes. Add the almonds, stir, and bake 4 minutes or until potatoes are tender. Remove from oven. Toss with the remaining ingredients.

12	ounces green beans, trimmed
6	ounces red potatoes, cut into 1-inch chunks
1	ounces slivered almonds
1	tablespoon canola oil
½	teaspoon dried oregano leaves
½	teaspoon salt
1	teaspoon grated lemon zest

COOK'S TIP: The lemon flavors develop as it stands. This is delicious served warm or at room temperature.

EXCHANGES/CHOICES
½ starch, 2 vegetable, 1 fat

Calories	130	**Potassium**	430 mg
Calories from Fat	60	**Total Carbohydrate**	15 g
Total Fat	7 g	Dietary Fiber	4 g
Saturated Fat	1 g	Sugars	4 g
Trans Fat	0 g	**Protein**	4 g
Cholesterol	0 mg	**Phosphorus**	90 mg
Sodium	210 mg		

Roasted Cauliflower, Onions, and Sweet Potatoes, PAGE 177

Roasted Cauliflower, Onions, and Sweet Potatoes

SERVES: 4 / **SERVING SIZE:** ¾ cup

1 Preheat oven to 425°F.

2 Place the cauliflower, potatoes, and onion on large foil-lined baking sheet. Drizzle with the oil and toss gently until well coated. Arrange vegetables in a single layer and bake 10 minutes. Stir and bake 10–11 minutes or until potatoes are tender. Remove from oven.

3 Sprinkle evenly with the salt and nutmeg. Wrap the vegetables in the foil and seal the edges. Let stand 10 minutes to absorb flavors and allow the natural juices to be released slightly.

- **3** cups fresh cauliflower florets, cut into 1-inch pieces
- **6** ounces sweet potato, peeled and cut into ¾-inch cubes
- **1** medium onion, cut in 8 wedges
- **1** tablespoon canola oil
- **½** teaspoon salt
- **¼** teaspoon ground nutmeg

EXCHANGES/CHOICES
½ starch, 2 vegetable, ½ fat

Calories	100	**Potassium**	420 mg
Calories from Fat	30	**Total Carbohydrate**	15 g
Total Fat	3.5 g	Dietary Fiber	3 g
Saturated Fat	0.5 g	Sugars	7 g
Trans Fat	0 g	**Protein**	3 g
Cholesterol	0 mg	**Phosphorus**	70 mg
Sodium	250 mg		

Brown Sugar Sweet Potato and Carrots

SERVES: 4 / **SERVING SIZE:** About ⅔ cup per serving

3	cups water
8	ounces sweet potato, peeled and chopped
4	ounces carrots, peeled, quartered lengthwise, and chopped
1½	tablespoons diet margarine
1½	teaspoons packed brown sugar substitute blend
⅛	teaspoon ground nutmeg
⅛	teaspoon salt

1. Place a collapsible steam basket in a large saucepan and add water. Place the potatoes and carrots in the steam basket, cover, and bring to a boil over high heat. Reduce heat to medium and cook 12 minutes or until potatoes are tender.

2. Meanwhile, in a small bowl, combine the sugar substitute, nutmeg, and salt. Set aside. Place the diet margarine in a small microwave-safe bowl and microwave on high 30–45 seconds or until margarine has melted.

3. Place the potato and carrot mixture in a shallow serving bowl, discard water, and spoon the margarine evenly over all. Sprinkle with the sugar substitute mixture.

EXCHANGES/CHOICES
1 starch, ½ fat

Calories	85	**Potassium**	360 mg
Calories from Fat	20	**Total Carbohydrate**	15 g
Total Fat	2 g	Dietary Fiber	3 g
Saturated Fat	0.5 g	Sugars	5 g
Trans Fat	0 g	**Protein**	1 g
Cholesterol	0 mg	**Phosphorus**	40 mg
Sodium	140 mg		

Lentils, Carrots, and Ginger

SERVES: 4 / **SERVING SIZE:** ½ cup

1 Heat 1 teaspoon of the oil in a medium nonstick skillet over medium-high heat. Cook the onions 2 minutes. Add the water, lentils, and pepper flakes. Bring to a boil over medium-high heat, reduce heat to medium low, cover, and cook 12 minutes. Stir in the carrots, cover, and cook 8 minutes or until lentils are just tender. Stir in the ginger, salt, and sugar.

- **1** tablespoon plus 1 teaspoon canola oil, divided use
- ⅓ cup diced onions
- **2** cups water
- ⅓ cup dried lentils
- ⅛ teaspoon dried pepper flakes (optional)
- **1** cup diced carrots
- ½ teaspoon grated ginger
- ¼ teaspoon salt
- ½ teaspoon sugar (optional)

EXCHANGES/CHOICES
½ starch, 1 fat

Calories	120	**Total Carbohydrate**	15 g
Calories from Fat	40	Dietary Fiber	3 g
Total Fat	5 g	Sugars	3 g
Saturated Fat	0 g	**Protein**	5 g
Trans Fat	0 g	**Phosphorus**	30 mg
Cholesterol	0 mg		
Sodium	170 mg		
Potassium	120 mg		

Black Beans and Tomatoes with Lime, PAGE 181

Black Beans and Tomatoes with Lime

SERVES: 4 / **SERVING SIZE:** ⅔ cup

1 Heat 1 teaspoon of the oil in a medium skillet over medium-high heat. Add the onions and peppers and cook 3 minutes or until onions are just beginning to brown, stirring occasionally. Add the beans, tomatoes, and cumin. Cook 3 minutes or until tomatoes are just tender, stirring occasionally. Remove from heat.

2 Sprinkle with the salt and spoon the lime juice and remaining oil evenly over all. Do NOT stir.

- **2** tablespoons extra-virgin olive oil, divided use
- **½** cup diced onion
- **½** cup diced green bell pepper or poblano chili peppers
- **1** (15-ounce) can no-salt-added black beans, rinsed and drained
- **1** cup sweet grape tomatoes, quartered
- **½** teaspoon ground cumin
- **¼** teaspoon salt
- **1** tablespoon lime juice

COOK'S TIP: Serve immediately for peak flavors.

EXCHANGES/CHOICES
1 starch, 1 vegetable, 1½ fat

Calories	140	**Total Carbohydrate**	15 g
Calories from Fat	60	Dietary Fiber	4 g
Total Fat	7 g	Sugars	2 g
Saturated Fat	1 g	**Protein**	5 g
Trans Fat	0 g	**Phosphorus**	100 mg
Cholesterol	0 mg		
Sodium	160 mg		
Potassium	380 mg		

Sweet Peas with Mint and Green Onion

SERVES: 4 / **SERVING SIZE:** ½ cup

½ cup water
2 cups frozen green peas
⅓ cup chopped fresh mint
2 tablespoons finely chopped green onion
1 tablespoon diet margarine
¼ teaspoon salt

1 In a medium saucepan, bring the water to a boil over high heat. Add the peas, return to a boil, reduce heat, cover, and simmer 1 minute or until heated. Drain, place in a serving bowl with the remaining ingredients, and toss until the margarine has melted.

EXCHANGES/CHOICES
2 vegetable, ½ fat

Calories	80	**Potassium**	110 mg
Calories from Fat	10	**Total Carbohydrate**	13 g
Total Fat	1.5 g	Dietary Fiber	5 g
Saturated Fat	0 g	Sugars	4 g
Trans Fat	0 g	**Protein**	4 g
Cholesterol	0 mg	**Phosphorus**	60 mg
Sodium	180 mg		

COOK'S TIP: The addition of mint "lifts" the flavors of the dish!

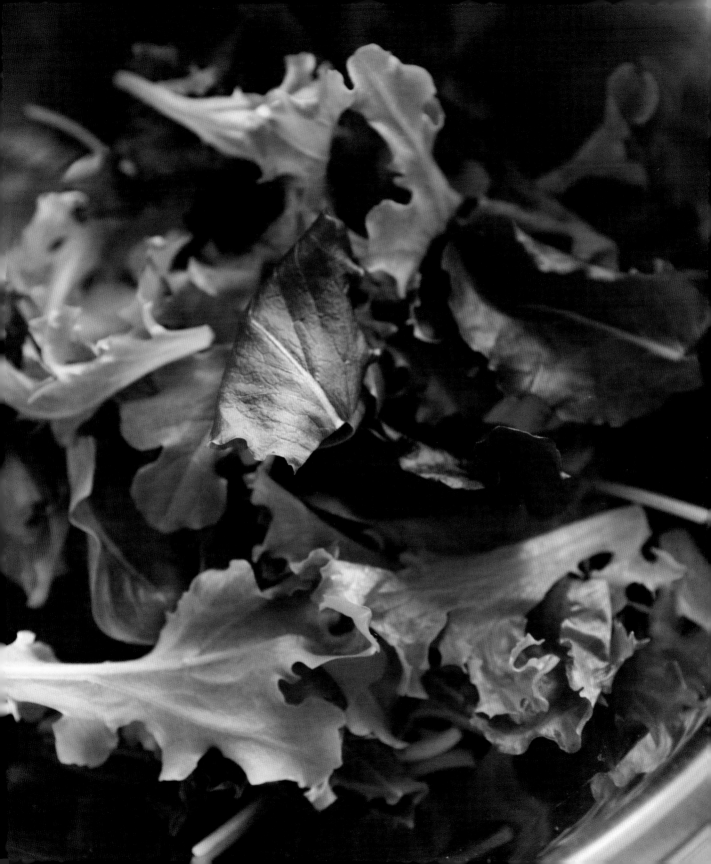

Desserts

NO-BAKE DESSERTS

Cereal Cookie Rounds

Apple Pie Phyllo Tarts

Toffee Almond Poached Pears

Berry-Sauced Pears

Grilled Pineapple Kabobs with
   Strawberry "Cream"

BAKED

Blueberry-Lemon Cupcakers

Cake Mix Cookies with Almonds,
   Cranberries, and Lemon Zest

Flourless Peanut Butter Cookies
   with Dried Fruits

Brownie Bites

Fresh Strawberry Flan

FROZEN

Strawberry-Peach Freeze

Pomegranate Peach Ice

Dark Cherry Freeze Pops

Peanut Butter and Chocolate Chip
    Frozen Yogurt

Cereal Cookie Rounds

SERVES: 24 / **SERVING SIZE:** 1 cookie

3 ounces sliced almonds

⅓ cup hulled pumpkin seeds

¼ cup sesame seeds

3 tablespoons low-sodium and 33% less sugar peanut butter

2 tablespoons canola oil

8 ounces miniature marshmallows (about 4 cups)

3½ cups crisp toasted rice cereal

½ cup reduced-sugar dried cranberries, chopped

1 tablespoon grated orange zest

½ teaspoon salt

1 Heat a large nonstick skillet over medium-high heat. Cook the almonds, pumpkin seeds, and sesame seeds 3 minutes until sesame seeds are golden, stirring frequently. Set aside on separate plate.

2 Place the skillet over medium-low heat, add peanut butter, oil, and marshmallows. Cook 3–4 minutes or until marshmallows are melted and mixture is smooth, stirring frequently.

3 Working quickly, stir in the almond mixture and the remaining ingredients until well blended. Place equal amounts of the mixture in each of 24 muffin tins and press down lightly to take the shape of the muffin tin. Let stand 30 minutes before serving.

EXCHANGES/CHOICES

½ starch, 1 fat

Calories	130	**Potassium**	65 mg
Calories from Fat	50	**Total Carbohydrate**	15 g
Total Fat	6 g	Dietary Fiber	2 g
Saturated Fat	0.5 g	Sugars	7 g
Trans Fat	0 g	**Protein**	3 g
Cholesterol	0 mg	**Phosphorus**	65 mg
Sodium	85 mg		

COOK'S TIP: Store leftovers in an airtight container at room temperature up to 3 days for peak flavor and texture.

Apple Pie Phyllo Tarts

SERVES: 5 / **SERVING SIZE:** 3 tarts

1 Combine the apples, water, and cinnamon in a small saucepan. Bring to a boil over medium-high heat. Reduce heat, cover, and simmer on medium low for 2 minutes or until just tender-crisp.

2 Remove from heat and stir in the remaining ingredients, except the tart shells. Stir until diet margarine is melted.

3 At time of serving, spoon equal amounts (about 1 tablespoon) into each tart shell. Serve warm or at room temperature.

1½ cups diced tart apple, such as Granny Smith
3 tablespoons water
¼ teaspoon ground cinnamon
1 ounce chopped pecans, toasted and finely chopped
1 tablespoon diet margarine
1 tablespoon sugar or honey
¾ teaspoon vanilla, butter and nut flavoring or 1 teaspoon vanilla
Pinch of salt
1 (1.9-ounce) package phyllo mini tart shells

EXCHANGES/CHOICES
1 starch, 1 fat

Calories	110	**Potassium**	70 mg
Calories from Fat	50	**Total Carbohydrate**	15 g
Total Fat	6 g	Dietary Fiber	2 g
Saturated Fat	1 g	Sugars	7 g
Trans Fat	0 g	**Protein**	1 g
Cholesterol	0 mg	**Phosphorus**	30 mg
Sodium	110 mg		

Toffee Almond Poached Pears

SERVES: 4 / **SERVING SIZE:** 1 pear half and 1 tablespoon sauce

1   ounce sliced almonds
1   cup water
2   ripe medium pears, peeled, halved, and cored
⅛   teaspoon ground cinnamon
4   sugar-free toffee-flavored hard candies (such as Werther's), coarsely crushed
1   teaspoon diet margarine

1   Heat a large nonstick skillet over medium-high heat. Cook the almonds 2–3 minutes or until beginning to lightly brown, stirring constantly. Remove from skillet and set aside.

2   Place the water in skillet, bring to a boil over medium-high heat, add the pear halves, flat side down, and sprinkle with cinnamon. Cover, reduce heat to medium low, and cook 5–6 minutes or until just tender-crisp.

3   Remove from heat and place pears in individual dessert bowls. Discard all but 2 tablespoons of the water. Return the 2 tablespoons water to the skillet over medium-low heat, add the margarine, almonds, and candies and stir to blend. Cook 30–45 seconds or until candy melts slightly. Spoon equal amounts over each pear half. Let stand 15 minutes before serving to allow flavors to become more pronounced.

EXCHANGES/CHOICES
1 fruit, 1 fat

Calories	90	**Potassium**	150 mg
Calories from Fat	35	**Total Carbohydrate**	15 g
Total Fat	4 g	Dietary Fiber	3 g
Saturated Fat	0.5 g	Sugars	7 g
Trans Fat	0 g	**Protein**	2 g
Cholesterol	<5 mg	**Phosphorus**	40 mg
Sodium	20 mg		

Berry-Sauced Pears

SERVES: 4 / **SERVING SIZE:** ½ cup pear slices and about 2 teaspoons jam mixture

 1 Place the pears in a shallow bowl or rimmed plate.

2 Combine the jam and water in a small microwave-safe bowl. Cook on high setting for 20 seconds or until jam is slightly melted. Stir in the extract until well blended and spoon over pear slices.

2 cups sliced firm pear
2 tablespoons sugar-free raspberry or sugar-free strawberry jam
1 tablespoon water
⅛ teaspoon almond extract

EXCHANGES/CHOICES
1 fruit

Calories	60	**Potassium**	100 mg
Calories from Fat	0	**Total Carbohydrate**	15 g
Total Fat	0 g	Dietary Fiber	3 g
Saturated Fat	0 g	Sugars	8 g
Trans Fat	0 g	**Protein**	0 g
Cholesterol	0 mg	**Phosphorus**	10 mg
Sodium	0 mg		

Grilled Pineapple Kabobs with Strawberry "Cream"

SERVES: 4 / **SERVING SIZE:** ½ cup pineapple and about ¼ cup whipped cream mixture

2   cups fresh pineapple chunks about 1-inch, (about 12 ounces)
1   cup fat-free whipped topping
2   teaspoons sugar-free strawberry jam
4   (6-inch or 8-inch) bamboo skewers

 Preheat grill or grill pan to medium heat.

 Thread equal amounts of the pineapple chunks on each of the skewers. Coat the pineapple with cooking spray. Cook on grill for 6–8 minutes or until pineapple is tender and beginning to brown.

 Meanwhile, whisk together the whipped topping and jam in a small bowl until well blended.

4   Serve kabobs with whipped topping mixture alongside for dipping.

EXCHANGES/CHOICES
1 fruit

Calories	60	**Potassium**	100 mg
Calories from Fat	5	**Total Carbohydrate**	14 g
Total Fat	0.5 g	Dietary Fiber	1 g
Saturated Fat	0 g	Sugars	9 g
Trans Fat	0 g	**Protein**	1 g
Cholesterol	<5 mg	**Phosphorus**	15 mg
Sodium	10 mg		

Blueberry-Lemon Cupcakers

SERVES: 24 / **SERVING SIZE:** 1 cake

1 Preheat oven to 325°F. Line 24-cup muffin tins with paper liners or coat with cooking spray and set aside.

2 Place all ingredients, except the berries, in a large bowl. Using an electric mixer, beat according to package directions. Spoon equal amounts of the batter into each cup. Sprinkle evenly with the berries (about 3 berries each) and bake on center rack for 16–17 minutes or until wooden pick inserted comes out clean.

3 Place the tins on cooling racks and let stand 10 minutes before removing from tins. Cool completely.

1 (16-ounce) box sugar-free yellow cake mix
1 cup water
1 tablespoon grated lemon rind
1 tablespoon lemon juice
⅓ cup canola oil
3 large eggs
1 cup fresh or frozen blueberries

COOK'S TIP: Freeze remaining cakes in individual snack bags for a portion-controlled snack or dessert.

EXCHANGES/CHOICES
1 starch, 1 fat

Calories	100	**Potassium**	10 mg
Calories from Fat	45	**Total Carbohydrate**	15 g
Total Fat	5 g	Dietary Fiber	1 g
Saturated Fat	1 g	Sugars	1 g
Trans Fat	0 g	**Protein**	2 g
Cholesterol	25 mg	**Phosphorus**	15 mg
Sodium	150 mg		

Cake Mix Cookies with Almonds, Cranberries, and Lemon Zest, PAGE 193

Cake Mix Cookies with Almonds, Cranberries, and Lemon Zest

SERVES: 30 / **SERVING SIZE:** 2 cookies

1 Preheat oven 350°F.

2 Combine the cake mix, oil, eggs, and lemon zest in a large bowl. Using an electric mixer on low speed, mix until well blended. Stir in the almonds and cranberries. Drop by rounded teaspoons about 1 inch apart on non-stick cookie sheets.

3 Using a fork, press down on top of each cookie to flatten slightly. Place on center oven rack and bake 8–10 minutes or until golden on bottom only. Remove from oven and let stand on cookie sheet 1 full minute before gently removing and placing on cooling rack to cool completely.

1 (16-ounce) sugar-free yellow cake mix
½ cup canola oil
2 large eggs
2 tablespoons grated lemon zest
4 ounces slivered almonds, toasted
¾ cup dried cranberries

EXCHANGES/CHOICES
1 carbohydrate, 1 fat

Calories	120	**Potassium**	35 mg
Calories from Fat	60	**Total Carbohydrate**	15 g
Total Fat	7 g	Dietary Fiber	1 g
Saturated Fat	1 g	Sugars	2 g
Trans Fat	0 g	**Protein**	2 g
Cholesterol	10 mg	**Phosphorus**	25 mg
Sodium	120 mg		

Flourless Peanut Butter Cookies with Dried Fruits

SERVES: 16 / **SERVING SIZE:** 1 cookie

¾ cup + 2 tablespoons low-sodium and 33% less sugar peanut butter

⅓ cup packed brown sugar substitute blend

½ teaspoon salt

¼ teaspoon ground nutmeg

1 large egg

1½ teaspoons vanilla, butter, and nut flavoring, or 1½ teaspoons vanilla extract

½ cup reduced-sugar dried cranberries

½ cup dried apricot halves, diced

1. Preheat the oven to 350°F. Place oven rack in center of oven.

2. Combine the peanut butter, sugar substitute, salt, nutmeg, egg, and vanilla, butter, and nut flavoring in a medium bowl. Using an electric mixer on low speed, beat until well blended. Stir in the cranberries and apricot. Spoon mixture into 16 mounds on a large non-stick cookie sheet about 1 inch apart. Flatten the mounds with the tines of a fork, making a crosshatch pattern on the cookies.

3. Bake until golden on bottom, about 10 minutes. (Note: they will not appear to be done at this point, but will continue to cook while cooling.) Let cookies cool on cookie sheet on a cooling rack, 10 minutes before removing from cookie sheet. Remove and cool completely.

EXCHANGES/CHOICES

1 starch, 1 fat

Calories	130	**Potassium**	150 mg
Calories from Fat	60	**Total Carbohydrate**	13 g
Total Fat	7 g	Dietary Fiber	1 g
Saturated Fat	1.5 g	Sugars	10 g
Trans Fat	0 g	**Protein**	4 g
Cholesterol	10 mg	**Phosphorus**	60 mg
Sodium	60 mg		

Brownie Bites

SERVES: 10 / **SERVING SIZE:** 2 bites

1 Preheat oven to 350°F.

2 Place the candy liners in 20 mini muffin tin holders. Coat liners with cooking spray.

3 Combine the brownie mix, oil, 1 tablespoon of the flaxseed, water, egg, and cinnamon in a medium bowl and mix according to package directions. Spoon equal amounts in each tin, sprinkle evenly with the remaining flaxseed, and top with the pecans.

4 Bake 20 minutes or until wooden pick inserted comes out *almost* clean. Remove from oven, place muffin tin on wire rack, and let stand 5 minutes before removing the brownies from the tin. Cool completely. When cooled, store brownies in an airtight container up to 4 days or freeze up to 1 month.

20	candy foil or paper liners
1	(12.35-ounce) box sugar-free brownie mix
¼	cup canola oil
2	tablespoons flaxseed meal, divided use
3	tablespoons water
1	large egg
½	teaspoon ground cinnamon (optional)
2	ounces pecan pieces, finely chopped
2½	cups fat-free frozen vanilla or chocolate yogurt

EXCHANGES/CHOICES
1 starch, 1 fat

Calories	110	**Potassium**	20 mg
Calories from Fat	60	**Total Carbohydrate**	15 g
Total Fat	7 g	Dietary Fiber	2 g
Saturated Fat	0.5 g	Sugars	0 g
Trans Fat	0 g	**Protein**	1 g
Cholesterol	10 mg	**Phosphorus**	17 mg
Sodium	50 mg		

Fresh Strawberry Flan

SERVES: 4 / **SERVING SIZE:** ½ cup flan plus ⅓ cup topping

3　large eggs
1　cup fat-free evaporated milk
3　tablespoons packed brown sugar substitute blend
1　teaspoon vanilla extract
½　teaspoon almond extract
2　cups boiling water

Topping

1⅓　cups sliced strawberries
1　teaspoon packed brown sugar substitute blend

 Preheat the oven to 325°F.

 Place the eggs in a medium bowl and whisk until well blended. Whisk in the milk, 3 tablespoons sugar substitute, vanilla, and almond extract until well blended.

 Coat four 6-ounce ramekins with cooking spray and pour equal amounts of the egg mixture in each of the ramekins. Place an 11 × 7-inch baking pan on the center oven rack. Pour the water into the pan and place the ramekins in the pan. Bake 40 minutes or until set and knife inserted comes out clean.

4　Meanwhile, in a small bowl, combine the Topping ingredients. Set aside.

5　Carefully remove the cups from the pan, and place on cooling rack for 10 minutes to cool slightly. Run a knife around the outer edges of the custard mixture, invert onto dessert dishes, and spoon equal amounts of the strawberry mixture over each.

EXCHANGES/CHOICES

1 fruit, ½ skim milk, 1 lean meat

Calories	150	**Potassium**	330 mg
Calories from Fat	35	**Total Carbohydrate**	15 g
Total Fat	4 g	Dietary Fiber	1 g
Saturated Fat	1.5 g	Sugars	14 g
Trans Fat	0 g	**Protein**	10 g
Cholesterol	160 mg	**Phosphorus**	210 mg
Sodium	125 mg		

COOK'S TIP: Be sure to use boiling water, not hot tap water, or it will take twice as long to bake.

Strawberry-Peach Freeze

SERVES: 4 / **SERVING SIZE:** ¾ cup

1 Combine all ingredients in a blender. Purée until smooth. Serve immediately for a soft serve or gelato-style treat or freeze and shave with a fork for a granita or ice treat.

- **8** ounces fresh or frozen unsweetened strawberries
- **8** ounces fresh or frozen unsweetened peach slices
- **¾** cup water
- **½** cup pineapple juice
- **3** tablespoons pourable sugar substitute
- **½** teaspoon vanilla extract
- **¼** teaspoon almond extract

EXCHANGES/CHOICES
1½ fruit

Calories	60	**Potassium**	240 mg
Calories from Fat	0	**Total Carbohydrate**	15 g
Total Fat	0 g	Dietary Fiber	2 g
Saturated Fat	0 g	Sugars	11 g
Trans Fat	0 g	**Protein**	1 g
Cholesterol	0 mg	**Phosphorus**	25 mg
Sodium	0 mg		

Pomegranate Peach Ice, PAGE 199

Pomegranate Peach Ice

SERVES: 5 / **SERVING SIZE:** ⅔ cup

1 Combine all ingredients in blender. Purée until smooth and freeze in an airtight container overnight or at least 4 hours to firm. If too hard, let stand at room temperature 15 minutes before scraping into a slush consistency with the side of a spoon. Freeze any leftovers.

- **1** (15-ounce) can sliced peaches in own juice
- **3** tablespoons lemon juice
- **¼** cup pomegranate juice
- **½** cup diet lemon-lime soda

EXCHANGES/CHOICES
½ carbohydrate

Calories	60	**Potassium**	120 mg
Calories from Fat	0	**Total Carbohydrate**	15 g
Total Fat	0 g	Dietary Fiber	1 g
Saturated Fat	0 g	Sugars	11 g
Trans Fat	0 g	**Protein**	0 g
Cholesterol	0 mg	**Phosphorus**	10 mg
Sodium	25 mg		

Dark Cherry Freeze Pops

SERVES: 4 / **SERVING SIZE:** 1 pop

8 ounces frozen unsweetened dark sweet cherries, partially thawed and diced, reserving any accumulated juices

1 cup fat-free aerosol whipped topping

½ teaspoon almond extract

1 Place ingredients in a medium bowl and *gently* stir until blended. Working quickly, spoon into four 3-ounce ice pop molds. Freeze until firm, about 6 hours.

EXCHANGES/CHOICES

1 fruit

Calories	60	**Potassium**	90 mg
Calories from Fat	5	**Total Carbohydrate**	15 g
Total Fat	0.5 g	Dietary Fiber	0 g
Saturated Fat	0 g	Sugars	14 g
Trans Fat	0 g	**Protein**	1 g
Cholesterol	0 mg	**Phosphorus**	20 mg
Sodium	5 mg		

Peanut Butter and Chocolate Chip Frozen Yogurt

SERVES: 4 / **SERVING SIZE:** 1 popsicle

1 Working quickly, combine all ingredients in a medium bowl. Stir until just blended.

2 Spoon equal amounts into 4 popsicle molds. Place popsicle sticks in center of each and freeze 6 hours or until firm.

1⅓ cups frozen nonfat vanilla yogurt, softened slightly

2 tablespoons low-sodium and 33% less sugar peanut butter

2 teaspoons mini chocolate chips

COOK'S TIP: For variation, place equal amounts in each of 4 small ramekins, cover with a small sheet of foil, and place in freezer until time of serving.

EXCHANGES/CHOICES
1 carbohydrate, 1 fat

Calories	120	**Potassium**	160 mg
Calories from Fat	40	**Total Carbohydrate**	15 g
Total Fat	4.5 g	Dietary Fiber	1 g
Saturated Fat	1 g	Sugars	14 g
Trans Fat	0 g	**Protein**	5 g
Cholesterol	0 mg	**Phosphorus**	70 mg
Sodium	60 mg		

Alphabetical Index

Note: Page numbers followed by *ph* refer to photographs.

Subject Index

Note: Page numbers followed by *ph* refer to photographs.

onion, 148*ph*, 149–150, 155, 166, 174, 176*ph*, 177
Open Faced-Egg Sandwiches, 42
orange marmalade, 30
orange/orange juice, 93, 155

P

Parmesan Garlic Spinach, 164
parsley, 169
pasta
    Blue Cheese Beef and Noodle Toss, 153
    Chicken, Pasta, and Spinach Soup, 62*ph*, 63
    Chicken, Zucchini, and Pasta with Feta, 129
    Italian Veggie and Pasta Toss, 134
    Sautéed Artichoke-Garlic Penne, 167
    Spicy Shrimp and Tomato Pasta Toss, 144
    stretching techniques, 4–5
    Tomato, Pasta, and Artichoke Salad, 111
    Zucchini Ribbon Feta Pasta, 136*ph*, 137
pea, 9, 103, 145, 182
peach, 197, 198*ph*, 199
peanut, 67
peanut butter, 25, 47, 85, 91, 186, 194, 201
Peanut Butter and Banana Toasters, 25
Peanut Butter and Chocolate Chip Frozen Yogurt, 201
pear, 98, 106*ph*, 107, 188–189
Pear-Cucumber Mint Salad, 98
pecan, 24, 69, 102, 187, 195

pepper
    green bell, 5, 51, 66, 126, 132, 151, 173
    jalapeño, 82, 84, 168
    poblano chili, 27
    red bell, 53, 84, 155, 170
phyllo dough, 187
Picante Quesadilla Wedges, 52
picante sauce, 52, 125
pimiento, 45
pine nut, 113, 133
pineapple/pineapple juice, 99, 101, 154, 190, 197
pita pocket, 56–57, 80
Poached Eggs on Chopped Toast, 40
Pomegranate Peach Ice, 198*ph*, 199
popcorn, 90
pork
    Baked Spinach-Bacon Casserole, 36
    Breakfast Pork and Green Chili Wraps, 20
    Grilled Pork and Sweet Potato Kabobs, 157
    Ham and Avocado Cracker Stackers, 92
    Ham and Cream Cheese English Muffins, 22
    Ham and Edamame Chop Salad, 76*ph*, 77
    Ham and Potato Skillet Quiche, 35
    Ham-Swiss on Rye with Creamy Coleslaw Topping, 54
    Minute Breakfast Tortilla Flats, 21
    Pork Chops with Broccoli Almond Rice, 156
    Pork Tenderloin with Chipotle-Orange Veggies, 155
    Pork Tenderloin with Pineapple-Horseradish Sauce, 154

tuna, 53, 83, 142
turkey
    Bacon, Lettuce, and Pepper Tortilla Wraps, 51
    Black Bean-Green Pepper Soup, 66
    Cajun Chicken Stew, 123
    Chili with Sausage and Beans, 152
    Italian Sausage Bread Shells, 55
    Sausage, Bean, and Carrot Soup, 64
    Sausage and Cabbage Skillet, 132
    Sweet Pea and Bacon Salad, 103
    Tomato, Bacon, and Cheddar Grits, 28ph, 29
    Turkey, Greens, and Strawberry Almond Salad, 72
    Turkey and Swiss Stuffed Eggs, 71
    Turkey Sausage and Vegetable Soup with Sage, 131

V

vegetable. *See also under specific type*
    alternative 15-gram recipes, 8
    Cheddar Sauced Chicken and Veggies, 124
    Chunky Veggie Egg and Bean Salad, 73
    Grilled Salmon, Grilled Veggie Quinoa, 143
    Italian Veggie and Pasta Toss, 134

    Italian Veggie Smothered Beef Patties, 150
    Jalapeño-Sour Cream Dip and Raw Veggies, 82
    Lemon Tarragon Veggie Potato Toss, 173
    Pork Tenderloin with Chipotle-Orange Veggies, 155
    Protein Hummus and Crisp Veggies, 60
    stretching techniques, 3–4
    Sweet Home Beef and Veggie Pot Roast, 148ph, 149
    Turkey Sausage and Vegetable Soup with Sage, 131

W

walnut, 70, 166
whipped topping, 190, 200

Y

yogurt, 32–33, 46, 128, 195, 201
Yogurt with Syrup'd Strawberries and Almonds, 32

Z

zucchini, 5, 129, 134, 136ph, 137, 150, 157
Zucchini Ribbon Feta Pasta, 136ph, 137